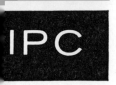

INTERNATIONAL PSYCHIATRY CLINICS

WITHDRAWN

APPLICATION TO MAIL AT SECOND CLASS POSTAGE RATE PENDING AT BOSTON, MASSACHU-SETTS. PUBLISHED QUARTERLY BY LITTLE, BROWN AND COMPANY, 34 BEACON STREET, BOSTON, MASSACHUSETTS.

SUBSCRIPTION RATE $18.50 PER YEAR. FOREIGN RATE $21.00 PER YEAR.

COMMUNITY PSYCHIATRY

EDITED BY

John A. Baldwin, M.A. (*Oxon.*), M.B., Ch.B. (*Aberd.*)
University of Aberdeen, Scotland

W. Malcolm Millar, M.D. (*Edin.*), F.R.C.P.E., D. Psych.
University of Aberdeen, Scotland

BOSTON

LITTLE, BROWN AND COMPANY

© 1964 BY LITTLE, BROWN AND COMPANY (INC.)

INTERNATIONAL PSYCHIATRY CLINICS

JULY 1964

VOL. 1. NO. 3

LIBRARY OF CONGRESS CATALOG CARD NO. 64-7779

PRINTED IN THE UNITED STATES OF AMERICA

Contributors

JOHN A. BALDWIN, M.A. (Oxon.), M.B., Ch.B. (Aberd.), Editor
Senior Research Fellow, Department of Mental Health,
University of Aberdeen*

W. MALCOLM MILLAR, M.D. (Edin.), F.R.C.P.E., D.Psych., Editor
Professor of Mental Health, University of Aberdeen

SHEILA M. BAIN, M.A.(Edin.), Dip.Ed.
Assistant, Department of Mental Health, University of Aberdeen*

F. DENYS BEDDARD, M.B., B.S.(Lond.), M.R.C.S., L.R.C.P.
Senior Administrative Medical Officer,
North-Eastern Regional Hospital Board (Scotland)

GEOFFREY E. FAULKNER, M.B., Ch.B. (Birm.),
M.R.C.S., L.R.C.P., D.P.M.
Deputy Physician Superintendent, Kingseat Hospital

JAMES G. HENDERSON, M.B., Ch.B.(Aberd.), D.Psych.
Consultant Psychiatrist,
North-Eastern Regional Hospital Board (Scotland)

JOHN H. HENDERSON, M.B., Ch.B.(Aberd.), D.P.M.
Physician Superintendent, Bilbohall Hospital

GEORGE INNES, M.D.(Aberd.), D.P.H.
Senior Research Fellow, Department of Mental Health
University of Aberdeen†

IAN M. LOWIT, M.B.(Aberd.), M.R.C.P.E., D.P.M.
Consultant Child Psychiatrist,
Royal Aberdeen Hospital for Sick Children

* These contributors are currently supported by grant from the Nuffield
Provincial Hospitals Trust.

† These contributors are currently supported by grant from the Medical
Research Council.

v

COLIN McCANCE, B.A., M.B., B.Chir. (Cantab.), M.R.C.P., D.P.M.
Consultant Psychiatrist, Aberdeen Royal Mental Hospital

IAN M. RICHARDSON, M.D.(Edin.), Ph.D.(Aberd.), F.R.C.P.E., D.P.H.
Senior Lecturer, Department of Social Medicine,
University of Aberdeen

GEOFFREY A. SHARP, M.A.(Edin.), Dip. Ed.
Senior Research Fellow, Department of Mental Health,
University of Aberdeen†

ELIZABETH A. SHELDON, A.A.P.S.W.
Psychiatric Social Worker,
North-Eastern Regional Hospital Board (Scotland)

RONALD A. Y. STEWART, M.B.(Glas.), F.R.F.P.S., D.P.M.
Physician Superintendent, Kingseat Hospital

PETER SYKES, M.B., Ch.B.(Sheff.), D.P.M.
Physician Superintendent, Ladysbridge Hospital

AILEEN TOUGH, M.A. (Aberd.)
Public Relations Officer, Aberdeen Association of Social Service

Preface

In such an ill-defined and theoretically confused field as community psychiatry, the volume of literature often seems to be inversely proportional to its worth. The only possible justifications for adding to the welter of words are to report the results of well-designed, valid research, and to describe the grass roots experience of that great army of dedicated men and women who, through every moment of time, bear the burden of caring for the mentally sick of human societies. This book attempts to portray, in an easily understood form, the accumulated experience of a small group of people who have developed and evolved over many years a comprehensive system of community services for the mentally ill in 3400 square miles of mountainous, sea-bound country in the northern part of the British Isles. Our rationale for such a book lies in the conviction that the work of this group is in many ways typical of other parts of the United Kingdom and in some important ways different from what may be found in other countries such as the United States. Thus, our aim is to describe the welfare society and the National Health Service, from what traditions of the deep past they have grown, and how they now contribute or fail to contribute to the mental health of the population they serve.

The person seeking help with emotional and relationship difficulties presents himself in countless guises to a huge variety of both formal and informal community agents. It is the singular merit of the welfare society that it has the unique opportunity among complex societies of coordinating and integrating the efforts of its formal agents toward the goal of maximizing welfare. The value of administrative unification or at least of de facto cooperation is patent in mental welfare. The extent to which this has been achieved in Britain and is exemplified in northeast Scotland is the subject of this book.

Part One, "The Development of Social and Mental Welfare," describes the setting of northeast Scotland, the conceptual framework of modern social welfare, and the historical development of health and other welfare services, particularly those most intimately concerned with mental health. The structural pattern is complex and not often familiar to the American reader. Still less familiar is the historical, evolutionary nature of the development of the services. There can be no apology for the reiterative emphasis on the past. It must not be taken as a nostalgic denial of the present, but rather as an expression of the real meaning of change in a stable society. It has to be accepted that things are not done so much because they "seem like a good idea," but because they are necessary, practical adaptations of past experience to present conditions. To describe the Health Service or the local government welfare services as they are now without reference to their historical origins would be to miss the whole point. That they could have been better designed for an ideal world is unquestionable, but they have to be made to work in a world that is much less than ideal.

Part Two, "The Integrated Regional Mental Health Service," describes some of the more essential aspects of the functional processes which the mental health service structure permits, as seen by those whose job it is to make the system work. The attempt has been to show some of the patterns of experience which the psychiatric patient may undergo, from his first approach to a help-giving agent, through the various kinds of treatment available to him, and thence back to the home and family to which he belongs. Inevitably, in a small book, much has been condensed. Only those aspects of community mental health practice have been selected which seemed at once representative and of special interest to the reader. If at times the writers seem to contradict one another, that is their prerogative. The practice of mental health in all its forms is still largely individualistic, for opinion and belief count for as much as hard fact; and practitioners must have convictions, even though based solely on their own experience, if they are to practice successfully.

Apart from descriptions of community mental health practice, the other area where useful contributions can be made is research. In this book no attempt has been made to indicate the scope of research in northeast Scotland; but for the sake of completeness, it should be noted that systematic studies in clinical, epidemiological, and operational fields are highly developed on a continuing basis. The intensive and extensive studies of psychiatric morbidity made possible by the psychiatric case register, and the neurophysiologic and biochemical work on schizophrenia are expected to pay large dividends as additions to basic knowledge and as improvements in service.

The title of this book hints at its theme, i.e., the integration of psychiatry and social welfare, which is regarded as one specific expression of the meaning of community mental health in British society. While it remains a principle of government that the welfare of the governed is a prime commitment, there can be no escape from its responsibility for community mental health. Conversely, medicine, and every other care-giving profession, whether state-run or voluntary, must accept the fact that, through its close relationship with the people, it mediates forces which advance or retard their mental health. In this sense, the integration of psychiatry and social welfare is a necessary prelude to maximal influence.

The invaluable assistance of the following persons in the preparation of the text is gratefully acknowledged: Alan T. Auld, J.P., Secretary, Aberdeen Association of Social Service; Margaret P. Buchanan, M.A., B.Sc., Ed.B., Principal, Aberdeen Child Guidance Centre; W. U. Henry, M.A., B.Sc., Deputy Director of Education, City of Aberdeen; R. B. McLeod, O.B.E., J.P., M.A., B.Sc., Headmaster, Oakbank Approved School; William McGregor Smith, M.A., Chief Constable, Aberdeen City Police; J. D. Taylor, M.B.E., Principal Probation Officer, City of Aberdeen.

Appreciation is also extended to Dr. Cecil B. Kidd, M.D., Ph.D., D.P.M., Senior Lecturer, Department of Mental Health, University of Aberdeen, for reading and commenting on the manuscript, and to Miss Maria Helen Ramsay and Mrs. Elizabeth H. Riddell for typing it. Mrs. Joy H. Baldwin kindly prepared the illustrations.

JOHN A. BALDWIN
W. MALCOLM MILLAR

Contents

Development of Social and Mental Welfare

The Integrated Regional Mental Health Service

xi

DEVELOPMENT OF SOCIAL
AND MENTAL WELFARE

Introduction

Many centuries of tradition embodying a multitude of influences are the heritage which contributes, at times it seems excessively, to the present British culture. Certainly a thread of continuity can be traced through history, yet the influences and traditions were never homogeneous, and there is not even now that kind of social uniformity which used to be fondly thought of as the national character. Indeed, the more intimate one's knowledge of Britain, the more surprising becomes the variety in styles of life most obviously expressed in a host of dialects, and even languages, in attitudes and beliefs, and in philosophical orientation. For 53 million people packed into less than 95,000 square miles, there is an astounding variation which persists in spite of every kind of massive force from urbanization, industrialization, and automation, to mass media, universal welfare, and total warfare. This historical diversity is still formalized in national distinctions in government, administration, law, social service, military structure, and many other organizational aspects of life. Apart from the jealously guarded national distinctions between the English, the Welsh, the Northern Irish, and the Scots, there are equally intensively maintained local differences down through every level of social organization to village, street, and family.

Against this backdrop of individualistic nonconformity must be set the major forces which both maintain stability and mediate change. Perhaps the very parochialism of loyalty and affiliation, which has its historic roots in long continued strife and national disorganization, provides the necessary condition for stability. Tradition militates against change, prevents mobility, and encourages acceptance of the status quo. Social change must be slow, grudging, and usually falls short of the optimism of the contemporary reformer.

That the entrenched injustices of the nineteenth century could not survive the tremendous pressures of the twentieth was not the result of twentieth-century events so much as the realization of social goals defined and worked toward for perhaps a hundred years. The established movement of labor found effective political expression in the twenties and thirties. Economic depressions had provided the conditions for success. Yet as long before this as 1911 the Liberal leader, David Lloyd George, had institutionalized the principle of social welfare in the panel insurance scheme. The war which followed the partial economic recovery in 1939 delayed, yet encouraged, the peaceful social revolution it preceded. The socialist government which followed victory in 1945 did not herald this revolution, it continued a process begun long before, planned in the wartime Beveridge Report, and already partially executed.

Since that time, consolidation has been marked by a series of measures like the Mental Health Acts, which have amended and improved various aspects of the welfare structure shown to be deficient. Social welfare is no longer a political platform in Britain, it is part of the fabric of society. Its goals cut across all party lines from extreme left to extreme right. Its principles are as inviolable as the United States Constitution, its practice so interlaced with the culture that it has become part of the social tradition, and to change it would be again a gradual, trying process.

In this part of the book, some of these facets of the social scene are indicated. It begins with a description of the northeast of Scotland because it is different than the rest of Scotland, and different than England, Wales, and Northern Ireland. In "The Integration of Welfare," the social welfare system and the National Health Service are described because, in their universality, they touch deeply this locality. The chapter goes on to recount the chief forces which have contributed to psychiatry in Scotland because in many ways these are quite specific and directly relevant to today's structure of community mental health. Lastly, some of the local social services are depicted in detail as the local interpretation of the national ethos. The third chapter deals with staffing structure in the National Health Service and with the associated problems of training and recruitment. Staffing structure is peculiarly British and an understanding of it is essential to appreciation of the descriptions of the mental health services in Part Two, "The Integrated Regional Mental Health Service."

The Northeast Region of Scotland

Scotland is the most northerly of the four countries making up the United Kingdom (Figure 1A). Although its area of 30,411 square miles is approximately 30 per cent of the United Kingdom, only about 10 per cent of the total population live in Scotland. The overall density of population is 174 persons per square mile compared with 790 per square mile in England and Wales.

The mainland of Scotland is divided into three parts: (1) the Highlands, mainly mountainous with scattered pockets of population along the coastal plains; (2) the Central Lowlands, comprising the main industrial areas with approximately 75 per cent of the population; and (3) the Southern Uplands, less mountainous and more populous than the Highlands.

Although Scotland lies between latitudes 55° and 61° North, the warm North Atlantic Ocean Drift creates a temperate climate. In spite of great climatic variations, it can generally be described as mild and moist in the west, and dry and bracing in the east.

The Romans knew the country, which they called Caledonia, as the home of the Picts. Though they conquered what is now England, neither they nor other invaders from the Continent were successful in subduing the Picts, whose origin is not certain but who were probably derived from Scandinavian and other races.

The Kingdom of Scotland was formed about the ninth century when the Picts united with the Scots, a Gaelic speaking race from

Ireland who settled in the Western Highlands and islands. Although the proportion of persons in Scotland who can speak Gaelic has fallen from 7 per cent in 1891 to 1½ per cent in 1961, there are still a few who speak no English.

In later centuries England made repeated attempts to conquer the Scots, and bitter enmity continued until the seventeenth century when James VI of Scotland inherited the throne of England. The country remained independent until the Union of the Parliaments in 1707. Despite the Union, the Scots have striven to retain their rugged individuality and even now there are those who advocate that Scotland should regain "home rule."

Not long after the Union there was a rapid growth of trade, best illustrated by the development of Glasgow, in the Central Lowland area. As a result this part of the country gave little popular support to the Jacobite Rising against the Crown in 1745–1746. On the other hand, following their defeat in the Rising, the Highlands were brought under the control of the central government for the first time. The English were determined to show their authority. After the Battle of Culloden Moor, at which the flower of Scottish manhood was cut down, chiefs of clans were shorn of their power, and families were broken up. Even Highland dress was proscribed.

Throughout the nineteenth century the industrial development of the Central Lowlands continued and was associated with a marked increase in population. These industrial areas were severely affected by the depression in the late 1920's and have never fully recovered. In January, 1964, the unemployment rate for Scotland was 4.7 per cent compared with 2.2 per cent for Great Britain as a whole.

GEOGRAPHY

The services which are described in this book are those administered by the North-Eastern Regional Hospital Board (Scotland). This region comprises the city of Aberdeen and the counties of Aberdeen, Kincardine, Banff, Moray, and the Orkney and Shetland Islands (Figure 1D). The mainland part of the region is approxi-

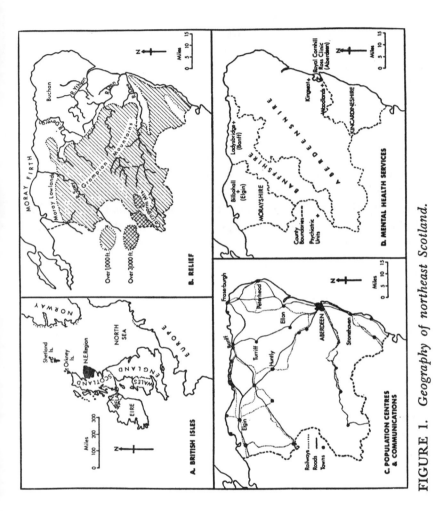

FIGURE 1. *Geography of northeast Scotland.*

mately 3460 square miles in area, or one-ninth of Scotland. It forms the eastern part of the Highlands.

The focal point or nucleus of the whole region is the city of Aberdeen. Even the Orkney and Shetland Islands off the northern tip of Scotland are within Aberdeen's sphere of influence since the air (daily) and sea (twice weekly) routes are directed to them via the city. Aberdeen provides the local daily papers for the whole region. These are important factors in maintaining the ethos of the area.

The northeast of Scotland can be subdivided into six natural or geographic units (Figure 1B).

1. *The Morayshire Lowlands* extend from Inverness to Banffshire. The soil is fertile and the elevation ranges from sea level to 500 feet where the Lowlands meet the Grampian Mountain mass. The countryside is well-wooded and farms are usually of 125–200 acres, large by Scottish standards. The main center is Elgin, a cathedral city with a population of 11,968, which is now the market town for the whole of this coastal strip. Along the coast are many small fishing settlements. Inland, settlements have developed along the river valleys and in many cases they are directly related to bridging and fording points.

2. *The Grampian Massif* lies south of the Morayshire Lowlands and west of the Buchan Plateau. It achieves maximum elevation in the Cairngorm Mountains in the southwest, where Ben Macdhui, the second highest mountain in Britain, rises to a height of 4296 feet. Above 1000 feet, permanent settlement is not generally possible owing to the nature of the soil, the harsh climate, and the lack of shelter. These rolling mountain ridges and high plateaus with their covering of peat and heather afford opportunities for the sportsman, nature-lover, and hill-climber as well as valuable summer pasture and grazing for cattle and sheep. The larger towns serve as market centers and tend to function as focal points of road and rail routes (Figure 1C).

3. *The Buchan Plateau*, fringed on the north by the Moray Firth and on the east by the North Sea, extends from northern Banffshire and Aberdeenshire to the limits of the city of Aberdeen in the south.

The two principal entrances or exits to this area lie in the extreme northwest and in the southeast. It is characterized by a landscape of rolling hills rarely rising above 600 feet.

4. *Kincardineshire.* In the north of the county the Grampian Highlands reach the sea south of Aberdeen, creating a historic natural barrier between the northeast and the rest of the country. Large areas are still covered with peat and heather, remnants of more extensive moorland. The coast is fringed with steep cliffs interspersed with small bays. South Kincardineshire consists mainly of a wide valley with fertile soil extending from the foothills of the Grampians to the low hills near the coast. Older settlements, small nucleated villages, are located where the valley abuts upon the mountain rim with newer settlements near the center of the valley, usually beside the main road and rail routes between Aberdeen and the south.

5. *Aberdeen City* is the third largest city in Scotland and its 185,000 people comprise about 40 per cent of the entire population of the region. It lies between the tidal estuaries of the rivers Dee and Don. Modern Aberdeen represents the symbiosis of two independent towns. Near the narrow Don estuary stands the town of Old Aberdeen, originally an ecclesiastical settlement clustered round St. Machar's Cathedral and King's College, which was founded in 1494. This old burgh with its winding High Street, its marketplace, and its Town House is today rapidly becoming an "urban fossil" in the midst of an extensive modern university building program. The other Aberdeen, on the north bank of the Dee, developed as a fishing and trading center especially with the Baltic countries and the northern seaports of Europe.

6. *Orkney and Shetland Islands* (Figure 1A). These northern archipelagoes, each consisting of about ninety small islands, are 376 and 551 square miles in area, respectively, and are impregnated with the tradition of Norse independence, the inhabitants still speaking with a faint Norwegian accent. In the Shetlands they are as close in spirit and sea miles to Norway as to any of the Scottish ports. The Norsemen viewed these islands as stepping stones and victualling

centers for their long-ships engaged in exploring the sea paths across the Atlantic to Greenland, Iceland, and America and on their plundering voyages to Ireland, the Mediterranean, and the Middle East. Viking settlements originally temporary winter quarters for boat crews, eventually became permanent when farming was begun and rapidly grew into townships.

CLIMATE

Although the average annual number of days with frost is lower in Aberdeen than in London, winter temperatures in the hills approximate sub-Arctic conditions for long periods. In valleys sheltered from the wind, temperatures over 70° F. (21° C.) may be recorded in summer, but these same valleys also act as frost hollows in winter. Snow falls on the high mountains from October to March and lies on the north facing slopes until June. In the Buchan area, exposed to the cold northeast winds, winter temperatures are low and snow falls on an average of 32 days each year.

Aberdeen, at a latitude of 57° North, is further north than any city of comparable size in the Western hemisphere and all except a few Scandinavian cities and Leningrad in the Eastern hemisphere. It is cold and dry in winter and in summer never reaches above the "warm" category because of cooling sea breezes. Nevertheless, with an average daily sunshine of 3.8 hours (varying from 1.5 in December to 6.1 in June) it compares favorably with Scotland as a whole (3.4 hours) and England and Wales (3.9 hours).

Due to their northerly latitude the Orkney and Shetland Islands have long hours of daylight (18½ hours) in the summer months. The climate is naturally oceanic and the average temperatures of both island groups are well above the mean for the latitude and only 4° F. (2° C.) less than London. This anomaly is due to their position athwart the stream of the warm North Atlantic Ocean Drift. On the debit side the islands have shorter daylight hours in winter and experience gale force winds about one-hundred times a year. Fog is also fairly frequent in summer.

INDUSTRY

By its very situation, Aberdeen City exerts a controlling influence over the industry of the region. In common with many areas in Britain where the railways are failing to pay their way, the rail system in the northeast of Scotland faces radical curtailment. Aberdeen is the terminus of the main railway from the south and from here it leads north to Fraserburgh, northwest to Elgin, and west to Ballater on Deeside. In the same way all roads radiate from the city like the spokes of a wheel (Figure 1C). Thus Aberdeen, in addition to having its own industries, acts as a distribution and marketing center for the rest of the area. Although the northeast is predominantly agricultural, there are also a variety of industries such as fishing, whisky distilling, granite quarrying, textile manufacturing, shipbuilding, engineering, food preservation, and paper manufacturing. Most of these industries, being typically small and family owned, are unable to compete with the larger industrial combines of the south.

Fishing

This is the other main northeast industry. Aberdeen is the largest fishing port in Scotland and the third largest in the United Kingdom. Other ports are situated every few miles round the coast, the largest being Peterhead, Fraserburgh, Buckie, and Lossiemouth. Fishing is no longer coastal; many of the larger deepwater fishing boats are now away from their home ports for tours of 14 days or more. The introduction of refrigeration and the modernization and mechanization of the boats have allowed them to fish progressively further afield, many going as far as Icelandic waters. With the development of these larger boats and the introduction of large-scale commercial methods, the smaller coastal villages have gradually deteriorated as fishing centers. Some of those to the south of Aberdeen have become more or less residential suburbs of the city.

Fishing is an important mainstay of the economy of both island groups, although the Orcadian tends to be a farmer first and a fisherman second, while the reverse is true of the Shetlander.

Whisky Distilling

Production of whisky is associated with Scotland and the term *Scotch* is known the world over. Total exports of Scotch whisky to overseas markets were 19.3 million proof gallons in 1958, of which 11 million gallons went to the U.S.A. Of the 94 malt distilleries in Scotland, 55 are in the northeast region, mainly along the valley of the river Spey. Many have over a million gallons maturing in their bonded warehouses. They use peat from the higher slopes of the hills for fuel and flavoring, pure water from the mountain streams, and barley from the local farms. Distilling, although such an important money-earner, does not employ many persons, only 20 to 30 working in any one distillery.

There has been a migration of skilled workmen from the northeast to the booming Midlands of England. Attempts to encourage new industry into the area are handicapped by the cost of transport of manufactured articles back to the main markets in the southern half of England. Thus, although the region has participated in the recent, marked nationwide improvement in living standards, wages in the northeast are substantially lower than those for similar work in England.

AGRICULTURE

Agriculture is an important element in the economy of the region. Although the northeast contains only one-ninth of the total area of Scotland, it accounts for almost one-quarter of the arable land. Its nature varies remarkably. In the Morayshire Lowlands the winters are so "open" that cultivation is maintained throughout the year and livestock are kept outside all winter. Barley and wheat are grown in the fertile soils. In the Grampian Mountains, settlement is only possible in the narrow glens between the hills. Small livestock farms, using the mountainous areas for summer pastures, attempt to cultivate a small acreage of oats and root crops for winter fodder. Farms in the Buchan area, although larger than those in the glens, are only slightly more fertile. In Kincardineshire they tend to be large and because of the shelter of the hills to the north and northwest, cereals gain in importance.

The islands have very small agricultural units. In Orkney they are of 25 to 50 acres, while Shetland "crofts" are from 1 to 10 acres. Egg production in Orkney is the highest per capita of any part of Britain and has brought great wealth. The Shetland farmer, or crofter, is also a part-time fisherman.

The northeastern farmer, like most of the inhabitants of the area, values his independence highly. This has probably tended to hinder agricultural progress. Although up-to-date equipment is too expensive for the average farmer, it is unlikely that he would consider sharing its purchase and use with neighbors. However, there has been a tendency in recent years to amalgamate smaller units into larger enterprises.

DEMOGRAPHY

Although the population of Scotland has increased steadily during the last 100 years, Table I shows that the population of the northeast region was at its maximum in 1911. Since then there has been an overall decrease of 6 per cent, while the population of Scotland increased by 9 per cent. Aberdeen (185,390 in 1961) is by far the largest town in the region. The next largest are Peterhead (12,502), Elgin (11,968), and Fraserburgh (10,460). The 31 towns with over 1000 population are classified as "urban." Changes have not been consistent throughout the region. Aberdeen has gradually increased in numbers but the Orkney and Shetland Islands reached their maximum in 1861, and have since decreased by 43 per cent.

Of the 90 Orkney Islands only 26 are now inhabited, many only by lighthouse keepers and nature wardens. Population density is 50 persons per square mile compared with 109 for the region as a whole. Shetland has only 19 inhabited islands out of 90 and a density of 32 persons per square mile. Between 1901 and 1951 the rural population of Shetland fell by 42 per cent while that of its only urban area increased by 29 per cent. Depopulation began at the

TABLE I. *Total population 1801–1961*

	1801	1861	1911	1931	1951	1961
Scotland	1,608,420	3,062,294	4,760,904	4,842,980	5,096,415	5,178,490
Aberdeen City	26,992	73,905	163,891	167,258	182,729	185,390
Rest of mainland	185,398	284,040	294,123	268,756	271,048	257,479
Orkney and Shetland Islands	46,824	64,065	53,808	43,498	40,607	36,552
Total northeast region	259,214	422,010	511,822	479,512	494,384	479,421

periphery of the island groups and, without doubt, isolation is a factor.

Depopulation of the islands is an exaggeration of changes taking place in all rural parts of the region. Movement to urban areas has been increasing. Over the whole region between 1861 and 1951 the urban proportion rose from 36 per cent to 63 per cent.

In the agricultural area of the mainland, recent changes have led to farmworkers living in larger communities. It was once the custom for married farmworkers to have a "tied" cottage on the farm and for the unmarried men to sleep in the farm "bothy" and have their meals in the farmhouse kitchen. When a worker left his employment he also had to quit his "tied" house. Now it is becoming more usual farmworkers to live in houses rented from the local authority and built in groups near a main road, while unmarried workers tend to live in the town or village nearest their work. This system allows a greater freedom of choice of employment for the farmworker and also brings him nearer the center of the community.

Rural depopulation thus presents as a migration from extreme isolation in the upper glens to relative isolation in the lower glens, from the lower glens toward villages, from villages to towns, and from the islands to the mainland. Since the last war, local authorities and central government departments have made efforts to arrest this trend. Undoubtedly, rural water and electrical power schemes together with road improvements have eased life in remote areas, but the last have also provided an easier exit route for the emigrant. Depopulation is further accelerated by lack of employment, Shetland having the highest unemployment figure in the whole of Great Britain—18 to 20 per cent.

The fishing industry presents another aspect of depopulation. Until recent years the numerous villages round the coast had their own fishing fleets. Each village formed an encapsulated community with little outside contact, and even some dichotomy within it between fishing and business families. Fishermen owned their boats which were handed down from father to son. Marriages were commonly between members of the same village, so maintaining the closely knit community. Certain surnames are found frequently in one village and seldom in the rest of the area. To take an example from the regional telephone directory, the surname *West* occurs 75 times. Of these, 31 live in the village of Gardenstown with less than 1000 inhabitants. The newer deep-sea fishing boats are unsuitable for the smaller harbors. Thus fishermen now mainly "fish out of" the larger ports—Aberdeen, Fraserburgh, Peterhead, and Lossiemouth. They still live in the smaller villages but travel up to 20 miles to join their boats, which they are now unlikely to own. These changes in the industry have led to the disappearance of the family tradition. As there is no other industry in the small villages, the younger generation are forced to go elsewhere for work, with consequent loss of young people from the coastal areas.

The population is also aging. In 1961, 15.5 per cent were over 60 compared with 14 per cent in 1951 and 11 per cent in 1931. This change in age structure is general in Great Britain. The proportion of wage earners to dependents has been decreasing and will continue to do so.

It is generally agreed that the population of northeastern Scotland is relatively static. At the 1951 census, for example, 86 per cent of the population were born in the region while a further 9 per cent were born in other parts of Scotland. Illsley and his colleagues (1) in the Medical Research Council's Obstetric Medicine Research Unit in Aberdeen have shown that, at the time of their first pregnancy, 89 per cent of Aberdeen-born women had mothers living in the city—indeed 34 per cent were living in their mother's home. Five years after the first pregnancy, 22 per cent visited, or were visited by, their mother at least five times a week and a further 40 per cent at least once a week. These figures point to the close kinship ties which are characteristic of this region.

Migration out of the region is increasing and there are also signs that in-migration is increasing although recent, detailed figures are not available. Between the census of 1931 and that of 1951, there was a regional population increase of almost 15,000. The increase of those born in Scotland was only 4000 compared with the addition of 7000 English-born.

DIALECTS

The speech of the northeast is a fusion of several elements still traceable in the place names and colloquial vocabulary of the people. The close affinity of Shetland to Norway, the use of Norwegian words, and the Norse accent of the northern islanders have been mentioned. The dialect spoken in Shetland can be distinguished from the singsong speech of Orkney. There are also several distinct dialects on the mainland. Though there are many place names with a Gaelic origin, there are few Gaelic speakers (0.25 per cent of the population compared with 1.5 per cent for Scotland as a whole).

The greater part of the vocabulary of this part of Scotland is derived from the speech of the north of England, and came north with the feudal system in the eleventh and twelfth centuries. This speech was itself a composite based primarily on Old English or Anglo-Saxon but with a large admixture of French, and of Scandinavian words brought in by the Danes and Norwegians who had first raided as Vikings and later peaceably settled in the northern counties. Also around this time Flemish weavers and artisans were introduced into the area to process the wool, skins, and flax of the countryside. Many words now in common use are taken directly from the Dutch. Thus a stranger to Aberdeen will find bewilderment when listening to a group of natives speak. Yet if he speaks to them he will find that they are almost bilingual, using what could be termed a "purer" form of English, but with a great loss of fluency. It has been said that the speech reflects the people, superficially somewhat grim, blunt, sardonic, and noncommittal, and yet beneath the surface durable, self-reliant, and sentimental in the better sense of the word.

RELIGION

The main religion in Scotland is the Church of Scotland which is Protestant in faith and Presbyterian in government. The proportions of the population belonging to any faith are difficult to estimate since no question of this nature is included in the national census. Admissions to the general hospitals in Aberdeen indicate that about 75 per cent of the population belong to the Church of Scotland. The Episcopal Church in Scotland and Roman Catholicism are the leading minority groups with about 5 per cent each. The strength of minority groups varies from one part of the region to another. For instance, the Plymouth Brethren are relatively numerous in the coastal towns.

REFERENCE
1. Illsley, R., Finlayson, A., and Thompson, B. The motivation and characteristics of internal migrants (Part II). *Milbank Mem. Fund Quart.* 41:217–248, 1963.

The Integration of Welfare

THE WELFARE SOCIETY

In Britain today, the word *welfare* is used rather loosely to cover a variety of statutory and voluntary services which have as their object the prevention or relief of diverse human problems. For example, *welfare foods* are nutritional supplements available at subsidized prices through the maternity and child health services administered by local government; *welfare benefits* are weekly cash payments to those whose earnings are interrupted by sickness, injury, retirement, or unemployment; *old people's welfare committees* are voluntary bodies providing clubs, meals, and recreational facilities for elderly people. So vast is the network of welfare organizations that at first sight the term *welfare* would seem to defy definition and to be beyond description.

Yet to those who are in frequent contact with the problems that these organizations have grown up to meet, two broad groups can be discerned: first, there are services that aim to put an economic floor below every individual; and, second, there are services which have as their object the satisfaction of needs of a less material but nevertheless important kind. Thus every person who is sick in mind or body and cannot earn his own living is entitled to claim certain cash benefits which are paid from either the National Insurance scheme, to which all employed persons contribute, or from the National Assistance scheme which is based on an assessment of resources. The people also have the following available to them without payment: medical care, skilled social workers to unravel their problems, welfare officers who can mobilize a variety of resources from housing to friendly visitors provided by a voluntary organization, employment agencies with staff specially trained in the understanding of disability, and many other services. The existence of these two groups of welfare services is a reminder, and reminding is still required, that human welfare comprises more than bread alone. It is sometimes too readily assumed that meeting minimum material needs, in cash or in kind, is the be-all and end-all of welfare—it may be a sure basis on which to build the upper floor of a welfare society but it is only a beginning.

The Past

Sympathy for, and action to relieve, the material and mental needs of others are as old as human society itself. Men have always in some degree sought to live in groups because they learned that certain fundamental and universal needs could best be met this way. Food and shelter, the rearing of children, and companionship could all be secured more readily by living in harmony with others; the disastrous effect on a family kinship of sickness or injury in the breadwinner was a powerful stimulus to the growth of simple welfare schemes to which, since none could be sure of immunity, all had to contribute. Out of these early stirrings of mutual help in time of adversity have grown our modern welfare organizations and through all their complexities and specializations there can still be discerned the same age-old motives that draw men together.

The history of social welfare in Britain has provided material for many books. Here it is appropriate to refer only briefly to some of the main developments in community action. The early social reformers recognized the outstanding problems to be the control of disease, especially epidemic contagions, the relief of poverty and destitution, the provision of safe and decent housing and sanitation, and the organization of adequate medical care. Planned and humane solution of these problems, at least on a national scale, dates from the early nineteenth century and reveals a truth which today is accepted and supported but which a century ago was perceived by the few: social progress is a product of knowledge and organization. A hundred years ago the machinery for collecting knowledge and organizing it into beneficial action was primitive; theories of cause were rife and untested—for example, epidemics of cholera were variously attributed to irreligion, destitution, drink, illiteracy, and faulty sanitation. It was the inexorable march of scientific knowledge and education that, harnessed to human feeling, brought about the program of social welfare that in the first half of this century produced what is now known as the welfare state.

The Present

In his *Report on Social Insurance and Allied Services*, published in 1942, Sir William (later Lord) Beveridge listed the five giant evils which stood in the way of social reconstruction: Want, Disease, Ignorance, Squalor, and Idleness. He showed how piecemeal were the attempts until that time to deal with these evils and urged the need for a unified approach to their abolition. Though the Beveridge Report was largely concerned with planning a new scheme of social insurance against interruption of earnings, its sweep was comprehensive and much of our present state welfare organization was inspired by it.

A brief account follows of the main services, first those provided by central government departments, then those administered by local government, and finally some examples of voluntary social services.

National Insurance

The Ministry of Pensions and National Insurance administers the scheme whereby all employed persons and their employers must contribute weekly payments, which are deducted at source, to the National Insurance Fund. On proof of (1) incapacity for work through illness, injury, or maternity; (2) unemployment; (3) retirement from work; or (4) widowhood, the contributor and/or his dependents are entitled to weekly cash benefits so long as the interruption of earnings lasts. Additional lump sum grants can be claimed on the birth of a child or death of a contributor.

The national Family Allowances Scheme, which is noncontributing, provides weekly cash payments for second and subsequent children.

National Assistance

Those who through disability have never worked or have worked only fitfully and therefore have not been effective contributors to the insurance fund can obtain, on proof of need, weekly assistance payments which amount to approximately the same as insurance benefits. But the bulk of the National Assistance Board's payments are supplements to those drawing benefits or pensions under the social insurance scheme. This apparent anomaly is due to the plain fact that many beneficiaries, but especially retirement pensioners, cannot subsist on the current rates of insurance payments. Any individual is entitled to apply for national assistance; if, on examination of resources and expenses, need is established, an extra grant or weekly sum will be paid. Most of the board's clients are old people but there are probably many in need who do not apply because they dislike asking for what they have not earned.

Employment

In every area of the country there is an Employment Exchange where vacant jobs and people seeking work can be matched. Employers are not obliged to use this service; unemployed people, who must register at the exchange before they can draw unemployment benefit, are also free to seek jobs on their own. An important section of the exchange is devoted to the special problems of men registered as disabled; a law passed in 1944 provided certain occupational facilities for disabled persons such as industrial rehabilitation units and sheltered employment.

Local Government Service—Housing

The foregoing services are national in the sense that policy and practice are centrally determined. Local government services, on the other hand, while subject to some control and advice from the central government, are not only administered at the local level but within limits can be varied according to community needs and wishes.

Thus the provision of houses to rent (public housing) is largely a local government service made possible by powers granted under the Housing Acts. Standards of size and quality are subject to central government approval and the cost of erection and maintenance are met by central subsidy and local taxes known as "rates." Public housing of this kind is a twentieth-century welfare service which, but for intervention of two wars and a period of depression, would probably have overcome the nineteenth-century legacy of inadequate building. In almost all areas, especially cities, overcrowding is still a severe problem and there is a long way to go before the welfare aim of a decent home for every family can be achieved. Increasing attention is being given to the provision of specially designed small bungalows and apartments for old people and much thought is also being given to the need for more imaginative planning, architecture, site lay-outs, and local amenities like play space for children and community centers.

Of the 27,000 new houses completed in Scotland in 1962, 19,000 were built by local authorities. The local authority has power to purchase any substandard house. Since the war this has resulted, in many parts of Britain and certainly in Aberdeen, in demolition of old slum property and replacement by new housing. Large estates with houses of the villa type have been built on the periphery of Aberdeen since 1945. As the available ground has been depleted and the demand for new houses continued, several blocks of "flats" (apartments), 12 to 15 stories high, have been built centrally in the city. In Aberdeen, as in most cities, it is not possible to keep up with the demand for new housing for people who are either unable or unwilling to buy property of their own. Thus it is common for young married couples to stay with their parents for some time before obtaining a "flat" in an old tenement property. The arrival of children hastens the time when they become entitled to a new "council house." Inhabitants of the other urban and rural parts of the region have less difficulty in finding suitable accommodation.

Wider Welfare Services

It has long been recognized that there are many human problems of such a complex nature that special welfare provisions must be developed. Primary emphasis has understandably been placed upon the problems associated with deprived children and each local authority is obliged to organize a children's department which, often in collaboration with voluntary agencies, is concerned with adoption, unmarried mothers, cruelty to and neglect of children, child guidance and behavior disorders, and other similar problems. Such services are by no means wholly devoted to cure or relief of deprivation; child health sections of the local public health departments are much concerned with prevention through, for example, education of parents on child rearing by "health visitors" (public health nurses).

Local government welfare departments provide many services for old people, such as residential homes, "home helps" who take over domestic duties while the elderly are disabled, home nursing services, and social workers who assist the old with a variety of problems. Those handicapped by physical or mental disability, including the blind, the deaf, and the mentally subnormal, are increasingly being helped domestically, occupationally, and recreationally.

Voluntary Welfare Agencies

There are many hundreds of these in Britain today and the services they offer vary widely in scope. Prevention of cruelty to children, accommodation for the aged, help with marriage problems, family welfare in its broadest sense, family planning, and recreation for those handicapped by the effects of poliomyelitis or chest disease are the aims of but a few of the larger societies. While some are organized on a national basis, others are confined to a few localities and thus availability varies enormously between areas. Cooperation between voluntary and statutory services ranges from quite nominal to very close; and, indeed, in some fields the local authority may delegate responsibility completely to a voluntary agency. More and more, however, there is a tendency to a kind of partnership between the two organizations: the advantage of the statutory service being its greater command of resources; the advantage of the voluntary service being its freedom to break new ground and experiment.

The Future

It is all too easy to draw a too perfect picture of welfare services in Britain today. Though it is probably true to say that a wide-mesh safety net has been strung below the whole population and more people are able to walk safely the high-wire of independence, two generalizations have to be faced. First, given expanded resources of money and trained personnel, far more skilled help and far better facilities could be offered for both the prevention and relief of welfare problems; and, second, more knowledge of the origins and nature of these problems is required—for example, far too little is known about the size and character of the burden of mental illness in the home. There are signs that the social sciences, starved for so long of the resources that other sciences take for granted, will soon be given greater power to explore both the theory and practice of welfare in the widest sense. With expanded knowledge and the means of applying it to human needs, society can look forward with confidence to an age when welfare and the good life are one and the same.

THE NATIONAL HEALTH SERVICE

It is difficult to define any coherent national pattern for the mental health services in Scotland prior to the introduction of the National Health Service in 1948. Legislation was centered on the protection of those unable to care for themselves and on safeguarding the community from the effects of contact with the insane. Mental illness carried a severe social stigma which, in addition to forcing a sharp division between upper and lower classes, inhibited sufferers and their families from seeking aid until no alternative was possible. Therefore, only a small proportion of those within institutions were there of their own free will. These institutions, as will be seen later, were administered in various ways, and the only statutory body with a general oversight, albeit in a limited way, was the General Board of Control. This body, originally set up in 1913 under the Mental Deficiency Act and later modified to bring mental illness within its ambit, was mainly concerned with all matters affecting the liberty of the subject and the interest and welfare of individuals, but one of its functions was to approve establishments for the reception of inpatients. These were of four main types.

1. Institutions managed by voluntary bodies. In the northeast of Scotland, the Aberdeen Royal Mental Hospital is an example. With a complement of 12 "beds," it was founded in 1800 as an offshoot of the Royal Infirmary replacing six "very good bedlam cells" in that hospital with which it retained a link in the shape of a joint corporation. It was managed by a board of directors formed of prominent citizens in the locality and derived its income from the fees of paying patients, from charges made to the local authorities for the rate-aided patients, and, to a very small degree, from endowments. It was permitted to borrow money for capital development. It was the teaching hospital for the Aberdeen University Medical School and, prior to the creation of a lectureship in psychopathology in 1938, the staff of the hospital conducted all teaching of mental illness. The directors also managed a country annex called the House of Daviot at Pitcaple and a small nursing home, not designated as a mental hospital, on the outskirts of Aberdeen.

2. Institutions provided and administered by the local authorities—the so-called "district mental hospitals." In the northeast of Scotland these were provided by Aberdeen City at Kingseat District Hospital, Newmachar, by Banff County at Ladysbridge, and by the Counties of Moray and Nairn at Bilbohall Hospital in Elgin. Aberdeenshire paid for the reception of patients at the Royal Mental Hospital; Kincardineshire and Zetland were similarly in contract with Montrose Royal Hospital, while Orkney looked to Edinburgh Royal Hospital.

3. Certain poorhouses with restricted licenses for the reception of mental patients were available which were also the responsibility of local authorities. Examples in the area were at Stonehaven in Kincardineshire and Maud in Aberdeenshire.

4. Private profit-making institutions which cared for only a very small proportion of the total inpatient population. In addition, certain patients were boarded out in approved homes.

The local health authorities, in addition to their hospital responsibilities, were also authorized to provide for the establishment of
psychiatric outpatient clinics at general hospitals or mental hospitals; to make arrangements for after-care; and, with the consent of
the Board of Control, to foster research. But although these powers
gave wide scope for action very few authorities seem to have taken
full advantage of them.

Motives for Change

Before considering the effects of the National Health Service Act
on the mental health services, it is necessary to survey the motives
which lay behind the new legislation. The first objective was to
provide health care without the necessity to meet the financial liability at the time of need, and furthermore to spread that liability,
not only in time but also according to the ability to pay. Some of
the burden, therefore, is carried by those in employment, the
healthy, through compulsory insurance, and a greater part by the
public at large through general taxation which collects from all,
but most from those best able to pay. Before 1948 the poor were already receiving health services at little or no cost to themselves at
the time of illness and it was, therefore, the middle classes to whom
benefit seemed the more apparent.

The second objective was to organize and administer the hospital
service so as to make it one integrated whole. Progress had been
very uneven and the better hospital facilities were to be found in
the more prosperous districts. By bringing them under one organization, it was hoped that inequalities and duplication would be gradually removed and replaced by a planned expansion dictated only
by needs. It was particularly emphasized that there was a need to
bring the mental health services into partnership with the other
services and to raise the status of psychiatry in the profession.

Finally, it was desired to set up an all-embracing national authority, in the words of Beveridge, "with the duty and with the power of
attacking disease as a national enemy." The Health Service is itself
an interdependent part of the wider conception of the welfare state,
used here in the sense of a society committed to protect the individ-

ual from the evils which stem from ill-health, unemployment, or ignorance. A national health service is impotent without the other elements of the welfare state, and the welfare state is inconceivable without a health service. One example of this interdependence is the purely economic aspect. It would be nonsense for a community to provide high cash benefits for disability without doing something to reduce the number of disabled. By the same token, it would be ridiculous to go to considerable trouble to prevent or relieve ill health without taking action to offset the social conditions in which disease prospers.

The National Health Service Act

In the administrative field, the effects of the National Health Service Act (Scotland), 1947, may be summarized as follows. The Secretary of State for Scotland, as head of the Home and Health Department, is responsible to Parliament for the National Health Service and for many other measures designed to improve the health and welfare of the Scottish people, including the welfare of aged and handicapped persons. Under this overall responsibility, the service is organized in three main divisions (Figure 2).

1. GENERAL PRACTITIONER SERVICES. These are administered through 25 executive councils consisting of both professional and lay members serving on a voluntary basis. They are mainly concerned with the appointment of general practitioners and their payment on a per capita basis. They are not responsible for providing or maintaining the premises from which general practitioners work but must satisfy themselves that such premises are of a satisfactory standard. They also have certain disciplinary functions but have no control over clinical practice. In the northeast region there are five councils serving Aberdeen City; Aberdeenshire and Kincardineshire; the counties of Banff, Moray, and Nairn; the county of Orkney; and the county of Zetland. The councils are advised by medical, pharmaceutical, dental, and optical committees drawn from members of these professions serving in their localities.

2. THE HOSPITAL AND SPECIALIST SERVICES. These are administered on behalf of the Secretary of State by five regional hospital

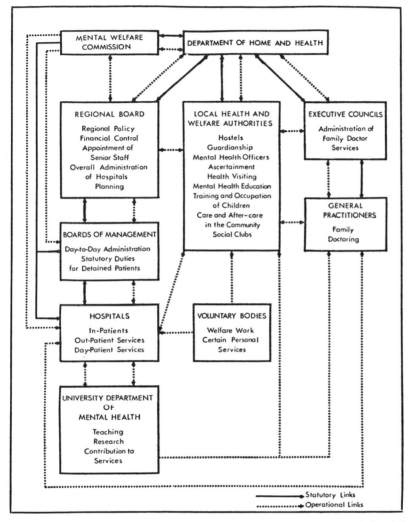

FIGURE 2. *Administration of northeast Scotland mental health services.*

boards and 84 boards of management. The latter are responsible for the day-to-day management, on behalf of the regional boards, of the 400 or so separate hospitals and institutions in the service, including mental hospitals and the hospitals which provide clinical teaching facilities. The regional boards are responsible for the planning of the hospital and specialist services, for settling questions of regional policy, for the employment of senior medical staff, for the general oversight of the running of the hospitals by the boards of management, and control of the regional expenditure. The members of the regional board are appointed by the Secretary of State after he has considered nominations from various public and voluntary bodies. The members of the boards of management are chosen by the regional board in a similar fashion. The members of both bodies serve in a voluntary capacity and include professional and lay people, selected for the personal contribution that they can make rather than as representatives of the body which nominated them. The Hospital Service is almost entirely financed from the national exchequer.

The North-Eastern Regional Hospital Board supervises the activities of 12 boards of management in Aberdeen and the six counties of the region. Each board of management is responsible for the day-to-day running of a group of hospitals. One of these boards is solely concerned with managing the mental hospitals and their specialist services in and around Aberdeen itself where the major part of the mental hospital service is provided, while two others have mental hospitals in otherwise mixed groups.

3.   THE LOCAL AUTHORITY SERVICES.   There are 55 local health authorities in Scotland. Their membership is made up of locally elected representatives and they draw their finance partly from rates based on the valuation of property and partly from the exchequer. Their responsibilities include the provision of health visiting, home nursing, domiciliary domestic help, the prevention of illness, and the care and after-care of people suffering from illness and mental handicap. The education authorities are required to provide school health services and special schooling for the mentally handi-

capped. The area covered by the northeastern region embraces seven of these local authorities.

In the field of *mental illness and mental deficiency*, the General Board of Control for Scotland, up to the time of the Mental Health Act, 1960, operating within the Home and Health Department, remained concerned with all matters affecting the liberty of the subject. They scrutinized documents relating to certification and detention; requests for discharge were considered; and, in the case of certified mental patients whose insanity was in doubt, they could arrange for the patient to be examined by two independent doctors. Under the Mental Deficiency Act, the board had the duty of considering periodically the case of each certified mental defective and of deciding whether he should be discharged or continued under care for a further period. The medical commissioners of the board visited all mental hospitals and mental deficiency institutions where they interviewed patients and looked into the conditions in the hospital in relation to any matter affecting the welfare of the patient. Some patients were boarded out in private dwellings and were visited and supervised by medical officers of the board. It licensed mental hospitals and mental deficiency institutions conducted privately outside the National Health Service and managed directly state institutions for violent or dangerous patients. The board's medical members and its senior staff were also officers of the Department of Home and Health and in that capacity they were concerned with the Secretary of State's functions in the mental health field so that in practice there was no divorce of the administration of the board's functions from those of the Secretary of State.

It will be seen that the Act of 1947 achieved a complete coordination of health services as far as the central authority was concerned and also succeeded in integrating the mental health services, especially the hospital and specialist aspect, with other sectors of medicine. Coordination at the local level has not been so easy to achieve, due to the division of the health services into three branches. It has depended on three factors: cross-membership between local authorities, executive councils, and hospital boards; coordinating committees, though meetings have generally been infrequent; and by

TABLE II. *Northeast region mental hospitals: bed complements, annual discharges, and numbers of staff, 1948 and 1962*

	1948	1962
Bed complements		
Aberdeen Royal Infirmary	5	—
Ross Clinic	—	38
Royal Mental Hospital	867	897
Kingseat Hospital	680	810
Wellwood Home	22	20
House of Daviot	130	130
Ladysbridge Hospital	225	225
Bilbohall Hospital	216	216
	2,145	2,336
Discharges per annum		
Aberdeen Royal Infirmary	40	—
Ross Clinic	—	246
Royal Mental Hospital	450	636
Kingseat Hospital	480	426
Wellwood Home	132	83
House of Daviot	100	28
Ladysbridge Hospital	50	40
Bilbohall Hospital	40	203
	1,292	1,662
Staff (excluding university and research staff)		
Consultants	5	10
Other Medical	16	24
Psychiatric Social Workers	—	6
Clinical Psychologists	—	4
Full-time Nurses	470	665
Part-time Nurses (shown as full-time equivalents)	41	33
Nurses (Total)	511	698*

* Part of this increase is accounted for by a shorter working week.

personal contact between fieldworkers and administrators of the three branches. It is probably the last of these which has gone further to achieve the limited degree of coordination which does exist. Table II lists the beds, discharges, and staffing figures for the years 1948 and 1962 in the North-Eastern Regional Board area and gives some index of the increased activity in recent years.

The Mental Health (Scotland) Act, 1960

After a few years of the National Health Service at work, it became apparent that legislation for the care and treatment of mentally disordered persons, for their protection, and for safeguarding their property and affairs, needed to be brought up to date. The existing acts had been subject to considerable amendment over the years, terminology was outmoded, and many of the underlying concepts were no longer in tune with modern attitudes, advances in medicine, and other facets of social organization, some of which had been brought about by the National Health Service Act itself.

The new Mental Health Act, while preserving the better features of the existing code, seeks to offer the mentally disordered patient the same ready access, without formality, to care and treatment as is enjoyed by the patient suffering from a physical disorder. The act makes little change in administrative arrangements for hospital care—the National Health Service Act had already brought about major changes as has been seen—but certain important aspects are worth noting. Particular hospitals are no longer designated as mental hospitals or mental deficiency institutions for the purpose of receiving mentally disordered persons. Separate provision is, however, made for state hospitals catering for patients requiring treatment under conditions of special security on account of their dangerous, violent, or criminal propensities.

Nothing in the act prevents a patient requiring treatment for mental disorder from being admitted if he wishes to any hospital or nursing home with the necessary facilities in the same informal way as a patient accepting hospital treatment for a physical disability. The procedures for compulsory admission of patients to hospitals or to guardianship are modified though with similar safeguards for the patient. The admission must be recommended by two doctors on the application of the nearest relative, or by the local authority's mental health officer if the nearest relative is unable or unwilling. The recommendation must be approved by the sheriff. A new independent central authority called the Mental Welfare Commission and replacing the Board of Control has a duty to protect the rights of individuals and can order the discharge of a patient from hospital if the commission considers he is wrongfully detained. They also advise the Secretary of State on any matter arising out of the act which he may refer to them.

The act made a much greater impact on the functions of local authorities (Figure 2). Their part in the mental health service becomes more important as the benefits of keeping the mentally ill or mentally handicapped patient in the community are realized and because of the emphasis on after-care for the increasing number of patients that are now able to return home after short periods in the hospital. The services which local authorities provide, whether as health, welfare, or education authorities, are now made available for the mentally disordered as for others. These include the provision of hostels or guardianship, the "ascertainment" of mental deficiency, the appointment of mental health officers, the provision of training and occupation for children under 16 years old, and in certain cases the authority to act *in loco parentis.*

Previous legislation did not define insanity but the 1913 Act defined several categories of mental deficiency, including the "moral imbecile." There was always considerable variation in the practice of certification and in the criteria used to commit a patient to a mental hospital. Thus it was exceptional for psychopaths, drug addicts, alcoholics, and impulsive epileptics to be certified as insane; whereas, in certain centers throughout Britain, it became a common method of disposal for seriously maladjusted antisocial children and young persons of average or above average intelligence to be committed as "moral imbeciles." It was the disclosure of this disturbing irregularity that led to the rapid discharge of hundreds of these patients and was a significant factor in the setting up of the Royal Commission on Mental Illness and Mental Deficiency.

No doubt with these anomalies in mind, the English Mental

Health Act introduced "psychopathic state" as a separate category of persons liable to detention if under the age of 21. It was defined as "a mental disorder manifested only by abnormally aggressive and seriously irresponsible conduct." Thus the hospital service was to take over the responsibility for many young psychopaths previously dealt with by the criminal administration. The justification for the policy is evident: that it is preferable for young persons who show antisocial tendencies to be identified and treated at the earliest point in time and not to wait until their behavior warrants a court appearance. However, it is doubtful whether the psychopath should be so sharply segregated from other forms of mental disorder. This doubt was in the minds of those who framed the later Scottish act in which the psychopath is not a separate category. Nevertheless it has now become accepted national policy that the health authorities should increase their provisions for this type of case and it is probable that within the next few years special "psychopathic" units will be set up for this purpose.

In both the English and the Scottish Acts there are more far-reaching procedures for the disposal of criminal cases where the accused is found to be suffering from mental disorder. Instead of a prison sentence, the offender may be committed to a mental hospital with or without precautions or security. Discharge may be conditional only on recovery, or by order of the court or the Secretary of State. Crimes of all severity, except capital murder, may be dealt with in this way.

It will be seen from these references to the treatment of the psychopath and of the criminal that a major shift has taken place whereby the psychiatric services rather than the prisons, borstals, probation services, and approved schools are expected in the future to treat the unstable offender. It remains to be seen whether this policy will prove successful. The special problem would seem to be that neither the modern mental hospital with its open doors, treatment of mild conditions, and short duration of stay, nor the community services, as yet rudimentary, are organized to meet this new demand. Many psychiatrists regard these cases as completely disruptive in present-day hospitals and are reluctant to admit them.

Conclusion

In summarizing this short statement of the administrative patterns and their development, the following points stand out as worthy of emphasis: (1) The integration of the hospitals into a coherent pattern, capable of developing in a fashion complementary to each other. This capability has not yet been fully exploited. (2) The improvement in the status of the mental health service by being put on an equal footing with other branches of medico-social service. (3) The acceleration of the trend away from the provision of mere custody toward active treatment—a trend which has been in evidence for the last 100 years. (4) The growing importance of the local authorities and the widening of their powers so that they can take advantage of the declining but still present stigma attached to mental illness. (5) The development of research and the increasing time given to teaching the subject to medical students and nurses. This is contributing to the development of a more enlightened attitude toward the subject on the part of both the profession and the public. (6) The improved opportunities of the mental health service to compete for the available, but still inadequate, national resources of manpower and finance.

An important problem has not, however, been wholly solved. Machinery has yet to be devised for the full integration of the numerous and highly complex agencies which can be brought to bear on the patient and his family. Given a solution to this problem, the administrative scene is well set for further real advance in the care of the mentally ill as they pass between hospital and community.

THE ORIGINS OF PSYCHIATRY
IN SCOTLAND

Present-day psychiatry in Scotland has its roots in the medical practice, laws, customs, social conditions, and religious institutions of the past 200 years. Before this time the condition of the insane was one of utter wretchedness since those who were not identified as witches, and hence devil-possessed, were neglected, starved, or otherwise maltreated. The repeal of all acts relating to witchcraft was achieved in 1736, although superstitious beliefs persisted until toward the end of that century. It was in Scotland during the reign of George I that witches were last executed.

In earlier times, and for those who escaped the witch hunts or the pauper prison, a statute of Robert I, in the early fourteenth century, laid down that the custody and keeping of persons of "furious mind" rested upon their relatives and failing them, on the justiciar or sheriff of the county in which they lived. The custody of those of "fatuous mind" became the responsibility of the nearest male relative on the father's side. The sheriffs, and many relatives, tended to abdicate their direct responsibility by paying for the consignment of their legal charges to private individuals or private madhouses which were run for profit. For example, in the late sixteenth century one burgh treasurer's accounts, in common with many others, contained an item "To ane man to tak a field William Dawsoun quha is beside himself and trublis the toun £8" (1).

The only monarch of those days who claimed expert psychiatric knowledge was James VI of Scotland and I of England who, in 1605, conducted an examination of a young hysteric accused of witchcraft and drew up a detailed report. The signs of witchcraft were not elicited and marriage was prescribed (3).

Philippe Pinel

With the decline of the influence of the Church in the treatment of the insane there was a steady upsurge of informed public opinion demanding more humane care and understanding and gradually they came into the domain of medicine. For Scotland the chief impact was to come initially from France where Philippe Pinel, philosopher, scientist, physician, and psychiatrist, was arresting the attention of the civilized world by his prodigious social and clinical labors on behalf of his patients. William Cullen, Professor of Medicine at Edinburgh University, visited Pinel many times and was himself increasingly concerned with clinical psychiatry in his later years. He wrote extensively on mental disease and was the first to employ the term *neurosis*. Among notable psychiatrists whom Cul-

len in turn influenced was Benjamin Rush, "the American Syden-
ham," noted reformer and one of the signatories of the American
Constitution.

Sir Alexander Morison

Pinel's pupil Esquirol, the first systematic lecturer in mental
diseases, likewise attracted many notable Scottish doctors to his
hospital in Paris, exercising a profound influence upon them and
their students. Sir Alexander Morison was such a visitor. The first
of many psychiatrists to become President of the College of Physicians in Edinburgh, Morison initiated a series of lectures in that
city and later in London, where he was to practice with great distinction for many years. His lectures, published in 1823, went into four
editions. He felt that the systematic presentation of psychiatric
knowledge to the medical profession was essential to its proper
recognition, a view perpetuated in the Morison Lectureship deliv-
ered annually up to this day.

Morison, not without personal ambition, drew up a plan for a
professorship of mental diseases in Edinburgh University. A patron
was found in a wealthy widow, Mrs. Coutts, who was one of his
patients. The Duke of York and other notables supported him and
the university was prepared to establish the chair. But fear of the
stigma of insanity aroused the opposition of other members of the
Coutts family who thought that their good name was in jeopardy.
It was not until almost 100 years later that Dr. George Robertson
became the first professor of psychiatry in Edinburgh—and in the
United Kingdom.

Morison was but one of a long line of distinguished physicians
who made outstanding contributions to psychiatry in Scotland. Psychiatry has thus been regarded as integral with medicine almost
since the inception of the scientific era of the profession. It does
not appear that the psychological schools exerted much influence as
they had done on the Continent. The common model of psychiatric
illness constructed by our predecessors was one in which the individual patient's mental disease could be understood as a bodily disorder, indeed as a brain disorder. So long as this model obtained,

psychiatry was within the fold of medicine. Later developments of psychologic and social models of mental illness were to place psychiatry in a less central position in relation to medicine.

The "Royal" Hospitals

The most notable achievement in Scottish psychiatry during the course of the late eighteenth and early nineteenth centuries was the establishment of the eight "Royal" hospitals for the insane and the mentally defective. These hospitals were constituted by Royal Charter and Act of Parliament as follows:

1. 1781, Montrose Royal Mental Hospital
2. 1800, Aberdeen Royal Mental Hospital
3. 1813, Edinburgh Royal Mental Hospital
4. 1814, Glasgow Royal Mental Hospital
5. 1820, Dundee Royal Mental Hospital
6. 1826, Perth Royal Mental Hospital
7. 1839, Dumfries Royal Mental Hospital
8. 1863, Royal Scottish National Institution (mental deficiency)

Before these institutions came into being, a few cells attached to infirmaries, gaols, and poorhouses sheltered only a fraction of the total number of the insane in pitiable conditions of squalor and degradation. For the rest it was a matter of bleeding, purging, and other tortures at the hands of the chirurgeons; scourgings at the hands of the officers of the law; ridicule by the public at large; or release by death from intercurrent infection, malnutrition, or suicide.

For the most part the new asylums owed their origin to the initiative of the medical leaders of the day, supported by men of substance and civic dignitaries. There was widespread concern for the mentally afflicted during the prolonged illness of George III, no doubt enhanced by the detailed report on his case history published in 1790. Even His Majesty was treated with scant respect and much brutality by his professional advisors and the public alike until the inhumanity of their attitude was brought home to them.

Legislation

By 1839 there were some 2100 patients in the seven Royal Asylums, of whom 1500 were paupers. However, despite the foresight and wisdom of those who created them, the asylums were often the centers of continued abuse and maltreatment and the first statutes in Scotland attempting to regulate the confinement and treatment of lunatics, the Lunacy Acts of 1815, 1828, and 1841, did not extend to them (1). The sheriff (a salaried Scottish judge) had wide powers under these acts to grant licenses for the reception of lunatics, to inspect houses, and to set free those improperly detained therein. It was also required that statutory books and registers of inmates be kept. These acts bore the marks of hasty drafting and there were many discrepancies between one act and another. Even the sheriff was comparatively powerless to redress injustices disclosed by his visits of inspection and many paupers, not required to be registered, suffered detention and ill-treatment within the law.

The condition of the pauper lunatic was to remain precarious for many years, indeed until the National Health Service Act, 1947. The Poor Law Amendment Act, 1845, placed the main responsibility, not only for the welfare of the pauper but also for his hospital treatment, upon the parish authorities, and in more recent times upon the local health authorities. Inspectors of the poor were responsible for lodging pauper lunatics in an establishment authorized for the reception of the insane, but the law was such that parish authorities could, if they wished, make other arrangements for their care. This could result in no action being taken unless the patient was prepared to pay for his treatment. Thus it was always possible to withhold treatment from those in greatest need. It was not until the early part of the present century that local authorities began to construct their own district hospitals for the reception of paupers. Many of these (of which Kingseat is one) were designed and built on the most modern and pleasing lines in a group of villas. In the mistaken belief that country air was good for lunatics, most were situated some distance from cities. Staff shortage and overall lack of finance soon vitiated the good intentions of the founders so that the lives of patients were far from privileged. It is of interest that the term *pauper lunatic* remained both a legal and a social reality until 1947.

The Reformers

While it is true that the medical profession played a dominant part in all these developments, a few lay reformers made their own significant contribution. It was Mrs. Susan Scott, or Carnegie, whose husband fought at Culloden with the forces of Bonnie Prince Charlie and later made his fortune as a merchant in Gothenburg, who founded the "Royal Lunatic Asylum, Infirmary and Dispensary" at Montrose and who may be regarded as the pioneer of mental and social welfare in Scotland (2).

A close friend of Mrs. Carnegie was John Forbes, formerly a Bombay merchant and banker, whose bequest of £10,000 led to the foundation of a new lunatic asylum in Aberdeen. His nephew, Sir Charles Forbes, Baronet, was further associated with these developments; the part he played can be seen to this day on the commemorative obelisk in the grounds of the present Royal Mental Hospital: "the worthy successor of his uncle in all virtues of liberality and benevolence with a munificence shedding lustre on the bequest itself, paid to the Government the Legacy Duty amounting to One Thousand Pounds Sterling."

DOROTHEA LYNDE DIX. Of all these reformers, both medical and lay, none can be compared for sheer impact of character, dynamic action, and range of effectiveness with that American social phenomenon, Dorothea Lynde Dix. Recuperating in Edinburgh from tuberculosis in February, 1855, having already made her name as the champion of the insane in Massachusetts and throughout the Union, she visited a number of homes for the mentally ill in the district. At once she was appalled and decided that the facts should be made known to the government of the day. The Lord Provost of Edinburgh was immediately approached. At first he was unhelpful and later became alarmed when Miss Dix took the first train for London. He could not prevent her from laying a detailed indictment before the Home Secretary, Lord Shaftesbury, the very next day. The Lord Chancellor, the Lord Advocate for Scotland, the Queen's Physician, the Duke of Argyll, and many others of high estate were worn down by her relentless logic within the next few days. It is scarcely to be believed but nevertheless true that this ailing, intrepid, and dedicated woman, who had never previously visited London and who had no contacts, within the space of two weeks extracted an assurance that the government would set up a Royal Commission of Enquiry forthwith. She wrote at the time (2):

> Today I have all business closed. I have two Commissions, one of enquiry, one of investigation in Mid-Lothian. This assures, first, reports into the condition of all the insane in Scotland. Next the entire modification of the lunacy laws, the abrogation of all Private establishments, the establishment of two or three new general hospitals, etc. My odd time I have spent chiefly in securing the interest and votes of members of Parliament for the Bill soon to be introduced . . . .

Voluntary Admission—the Commissioners in Lunacy

In April, the Royal Commission was set up and all the reforms she demanded were realized. The findings of the commission led to the passing of the Lunacy (Scotland) Act of 1857 which revolutionized the care and treatment of the mentally ill in Scotland. This act was to remain the principal legal instrument for the reception, detention, treatment, and supervision of the insane until superceded 103 years later by the Mental Health (Scotland) Act of 1960. One historic feature of the Act of 1857 was that it made possible the admission of voluntary patients to asylums, a provision that did not appear in the corresponding English Act until 1930.

The 1857 act also created a Board of Commissioners in Lunacy to take over the superintendence of the insane in Scotland, until then the responsibility of the local sheriffs, and to visit and report on all houses, licensed or otherwise, which might contain lunatic persons. Another feature of the act related to the disposal of criminals in whom a plea of insanity had been sustained. These patients were to "be detained during Her Majesty's pleasure." Medical and legal concern for the mentally ill criminal has always been a feature of Scottish justice, and was further demonstrated by the introduction

at the turn of the century of the concept of "diminished responsibility" as mitigation in serious crimes, a concept that was not
adopted in English law until the Homicide Act of 1957.

The Lunacy (Scotland) Act of 1862 simplified the procedure for
admission of voluntary patients but it remained too cumbersome
to be much used. In part this may have been a deliberate attempt
to place obstacles in the way of paupers who might find that life in
an asylum was to be preferred to life outside. The act also allowed
for the early discharge of selected patients on probation and so gave
the patient a chance to test his fitness to adjust himself to the
community before final discharge. This system remains operative
today.

Further strengthening of the powers of the board of commissioners was given in respect of certification, detention, and supervision of patients by the Act of 1866, which also further simplified the
procedure for voluntary admission. However, it was not until the
Lunacy and Mental Deficiency Act of 1913, which replaced the
Board of Commissioners with the General Board of Control, that
voluntary patients were admitted in significant numbers. A patient
could be received into an asylum as a voluntary boarder upon his
own written application to the medical superintendent, pending
the consent of the board of control. The patient could discharge
himself on giving three days' notice in writing.

The Guardianship System

It may be thought that many of our current concepts in psychiatry are recent inventions. Reference to history sets the record
straight. The policy of "open doors" was commonplace in the latter
half of the nineteenth century throughout Great Britain and the
example of Bilbohall in 1878 was by no means an exception for the
northeast of Scotland (see pages 617–634). Similarly, the notion of
"community care" was foreshadowed by an act of 1845 promoted by
Lord Shaftesbury which ensured the supervision of suitable mental
patients under guardianship. In 1857 the system came under the
board of commissioners and patients were "boarded out" in many
parts of the country, including the Western Isles. To this day there

are families—mostly in rural areas—that for many generations have played their part in preserving this tradition. Homes were inspected and guardians interviewed and selected. They were modestly remunerated. For the most part, patients who were placed in guardianship in this system were either defectives or schizophrenics. Scotland partly repaid the debt it owed to Massachusetts for the priceless gift of Dorothea Lynde Dix when the Scottish system of boarding out was adopted by that state in 1885.

Adolf Meyer

The Scottish-American *entente,* so firmly established by Rush and Dorothea Dix, has been continued with mutual profit until the present. Adolf Meyer studied for a time in Edinburgh, made many friends there, and cultivated these friendships throughout the rest of his life. He was much impressed by the serious-minded Scottish physicians and by the religious and philosophic climate. The Swiss, Meyer, like the Scots, had sprung from Calvinistic origins. Perhaps the common world of ideas had much to do with the innumerable visits paid by Scottish psychiatrists to the Meyerian mecca at Baltimore. One of the earliest visitors was Charles Macfie Campbell who later became professor of psychiatry at Harvard. He was followed soon after by David (now Sir David) Kennedy Henderson, first at the New York Psychiatric Institute and then at the Henry Phipps Clinic, where he was for a time Meyer's first assistant. Meyerian psychobiology was imported to Scotland when Henderson returned as physician superintendent at Glasgow Royal Mental Hospital, where he and R. D. Gillespie wrote their famous textbook, which is still a standard work in its ninth edition and still based on Meyerian concepts. Many of Henderson's pupils made the pilgrimage to Phipps, both in Meyer's day and later. Some, like D. E. Cameron, remained in America, but most returned to occupy positions of academic and clinical distinction in Britain.

Conclusion

One has the impression that the characteristic features of Scottish personality, professionalism, and scholarship are reflected in the psychiatric achievements of the past two centuries and beyond. There is a certain "canny" skepticism derived partly from the religious tradition of Presbyterian doubt and partly from the related philosophic tradition of Hume, its agnostic counterpart. Skepticism, empiricism, and the inescapably psychologic nature of "necessary connexions" combined in a particularly fruitful approach to "human nature."

The simple humanity among the physicians of the past derived from first-hand experience of early privations and disease in themselves or those close to them. Social and economic privilege were less often the spurs to achievement than were privations placed in a context of almost compulsive educational ambition. This veneration of learning resulted in the Scottish education and medicine that were unequalled in their day. The consistent reference to hard facts of common perception and experience, as expressed pithily in the idiom, "facts are chiels that winna ding" (freely translated: "facts are beings that don't ring hollow"), contributed to an intellectual climate in which there was no room for insubstantial theories and speculations. There was a ready acceptance of advances that were tangible and for this reason the anatomical and physiologic formulations were preferred to the purely psychologic. Above all, there was the concern for the individual patient, not only as the repository of all natural secrets that scientific activities attempt to explore, but also as another mortal whose suffering must be relieved.

All these varied factors acting and interacting within the historic process are to be discerned in the many social and professional institutions obtaining today. The concepts of welfare, medical and social insurance, community tolerance of the mentally ill, the indivisible nature of medicine and of the patient which is its concern, and many others, have now come to be embodied in laws and customs of which the National Health Service and the Mental Health Act are but two examples. The emancipation of the mental hospital from stigma, the shift in emphasis from institutional to community care, the removal of restrictions upon admission to hospital for treatment, and the intensified concern for other deviants such as the criminal, the delinquent, the unemployed, and the indigent all maintain that continuity with the better features of tradition without which true progress cannot be achieved.

SOME SOCIAL WELFARE SERVICES
RELATED TO MENTAL HEALTH

In the space available it is impossible to review comprehensively the vast array of social services which can be brought to bear, however indirectly, on the mental welfare of the community. A few of those which the reader may find most pertinent to his understanding of British social welfare in general and which he may compare with their counterparts closer to hand have been selected for detailed description. Since the relationship of the social services with the mental health services as such is often not direct, the former are also most appropriately considered at this point. For instance, though psychiatric services for children are relatively undeveloped in the region, it would be erroneous to assume that the welfare society lacked appreciation of the needs of its youth. Children's departments have already been mentioned, but the whole structure of the educational system and its integral health services is a vital service for mental welfare. Similarly, the probation service and the approved school system are counterparts to both law enforcement and education which have direct responsibility for the essentially mental health problem of delinquency.

Because the welfare society tends to be regarded as a matter of state and statute, it is often assumed that the spontaneous growth of philanthropic voluntary social service becomes stunted and sterile. It is important, therefore, that the integrative character of the role of the welfare society should be clarified from the outset. Here only an overall picture is given. Some voluntary services which are specifically orientated toward the mental health service are more appropriately considered in relation to their role as adjuncts to the mental health services.

Education

The tradition of education for the young in Aberdeen long antedated the introduction of state education in 1872. By 1833 there were 37 schools with 3664 pupils, many of whom were receiving free education.

The first school board in Aberdeen was appointed in 1873 and took over the central administration of nearly all the private schools in the city. Scotland has always had a reputation for a serious and enthusiastic approach to education, and the nineteenth-century pioneers in the northeast seem to have had more foresight than the authorities of today. The demand for teachers, which was bound to be created by the advent of state education, was foreseen by the Church of Scotland and the Free Church which set up colleges that produced teachers for the local schools. This was the framework from which the modern system grew.

Public education in Scotland today is administered locally by the various education authorities (county or city councils) and centrally by the Secretary of State for Scotland acting through the Scottish Education Department. There are also a few private fee-paying schools. All children between the ages of 5 and 15 must attend school unless they are medically unfit to do so. It is intended to raise the minimum age of leaving school to 16 in 1971. Outside Aberdeen, most schools are primary (children of 5 to 12 years) and in the rural areas most of these have only one or two teachers. With rural depopulation and the present trend toward centralization, many of these small schools are being closed, usually in the face of spirited local opposition. Thus children grow up accustomed to urban life during the week and rural life on the weekend. They naturally look for urban employment on leaving school.

After a common test of ability (the "eleven plus"), children go on from primary schools to either a secondary or a senior secondary school and specialize according to their abilities and aptitudes. Those fit are encouraged to sit for the Aberdeen Secondary Certificate (at about age 15) which leads to a chance of a better job on leaving school. In 1959 a new fourth-year course was introduced. The main provision in the senior secondary schools is for five years and leads to the Higher Leaving Certificate which is necessary for university entrance and for admission to various colleges and professional training.

The proportion of children who leave at the minimum age of

15 years is 67 per cent for the whole of Scotland. They may continue their education by attending evening or day release classes connected with their employment. It is rare in this area for a child to continue at school beyond the age of 18. Local authority grants, graded according to parents' income, are available to all children who continue in full-time education beyond the minimum age of leaving school.

Most primary education in the city is conducted in mixed classes and all the local authority secondary schools are coeducational, although boys and girls are taught in separate classes. Of the three senior secondary schools, one is exclusively for boys, another exclusively for girls, and the third is coeducational although individual classes are of one sex. During 1961–1962 the average attendance at schools was 94.13 per cent. About 20 per cent of the school population is supplied with school meals and 92.54 per cent take the free supply of milk every day.

HANDICAPPED CHILDREN. The education of physically and mentally handicapped children is provided at Beechwood School which was opened in 1954, and at an occupation center. The building and equipping of the section for physically handicapped pupils at Beechwood was completed in 1955 and the medical auxiliary staff was provided in the following year. Until a voluntary body opened a residential home for trainable but ineducable children just outside Aberdeen, there was no residential provision for such children.

The education authority employs a psychologist whose duties are mainly with backward children in primary schools. In addition, however, children in special and secondary schools are examined and advice is given.

CHILD GUIDANCE SERVICE. A child guidance center was opened by the local education authority in 1951, the functions of which are:

1. *Preventive.* An advisory service to parents, teachers, administrators and others concerned with children.
2. *Therapeutic.* Children showing evidence of social or emotional

disturbance are assisted along with their parents to reach improved adjustment in personal relationships and behavior.
3. *Educative.* For individual pupils who are not progressing scholastically in accordance with their potential, guidance is offered to the schools and in some cases the child guidance service provides remedial teaching in reading, spelling, or arithmetic.

The full-time staff consists of five psychologists, one of whom is administrative director, one remedial teacher, and one social worker. Another social worker attends half-time. Two psychiatrists give one session each week, and a speech therapist gives two sessions per week.

The problems dealt with consist of the following: specific learning difficulties, 23 per cent of cases; behavior disorders (including delinquency), 20 per cent; general backwardness, 17 per cent; adjustment problems, 11 per cent; habit disorder and emotional disturbance, 8 per cent each; personality disorders, 4 per cent. In the remaining 9 per cent, advice only is sought. Some 400 to 450 children are seen annually.

Seventy-five per cent of referrals are from educational sources, 9 per cent directly from parents, 7 per cent from medical sources, 5 per cent from probation, and 4 per cent from other sources.

The child guidance service is primarily a school service and therefore frequent school visitation is undertaken for discussion of individual pupils who are in need of help, guidance, or better understanding. Attempts are made to include the class teacher in the team where possible. Teachers are also given guidance in the detection of signs in pupils which may indicate a need for further investigation.

The center is specially equipped to provide safe outlets for emotional expression and activity. Children attend for a weekly period alone with the psychologist, or in small groups, to work out their problems. Play of diverse kinds (aggressive, imaginative, constructive, and social) is engaged in according to need.

Northeast Scottish reserve tends to control emotional expression. Many parents are undemonstrative and children have to learn early to control their emotions. There is also considerable drive toward educational achievement. The pressure, both to exhibit adult restraint and to achieve scholastically, places a strain on sensitive children. It is not surprising, therefore, that they frequently show symptoms of anxiety, due to a vague feeling of having failed to come up to the standards tacitly or openly expected of them by their parents.

SPEECH THERAPY. The education authority operates a speech therapy department which had ten therapists in 1962, and there are seven regional clinics throughout Aberdeen. One of these is in Beechwood School for mentally and physically handicapped children, where a full-time speech therapist is employed. Another has part-time duties in the child guidance center working with children referred by the principal psychologist, and two periods per week are given over to cases in the Royal Aberdeen Hospital for Sick Children.

Cases of speech disorders in schoolchildren and preschoolchildren are referred to the superintendent of speech therapy by head teachers, doctors, speech training teachers and members of the school health service. Twice yearly, speech therapists undertake a survey of new entrants into schools in the infant departments. These are carried out six months after the children start school.

There is close cooperation between the speech therapy department; the ear, nose, and throat and the orthodontic departments; and the child psychiatric clinic at the children's hospital. To meet the needs of children under five, referred as a result of retarded speech or incipient stammer, play therapy groups are conducted.

There are 13 teachers of speech education and drama who visit all the schools including the Pre-nursing College and the Commercial College. Classes in mime, movement, and creative dramatics are given at the school for the deaf, Beechwood Special School, and Rubislaw Occupation Center.

Probation Service

The probation service is a local government provision in Scotland, though like most social improvements it had its origins in voluntary work. To trace the development of the probation service in the northeast we must first look briefly at its origins in Great Britain as a whole. In conception, probation was a means of practical experiment rather than the outcome of clearly defined philosophic principles. The aim was to find some satisfactory alternative to the harshness of imprisonment.

The first "modern" experiment in probation took place at the Warwickshire Quarter Sessions in 1820. Certain young offenders were released after a nominal day's imprisonment on the condition that they returned to their parents or masters who were to supervise them. Supervision of offenders was carried further when, in 1876, the Church of England Temperance Society accepted the challenge of a printer who wrote to the society, enclosing five shillings with which to start a fund to assist offenders. Thus the first police court missionary was appointed. By 1900 there were 100 men and 19 women missionaries working in the courts of London.

In this way "the legal and religious approaches converged towards the conception of probation as we know it today; the conditional release of an offender under the supervision of a person attached to the court, who accepts the responsibility of helping him to make good" (4).

With the Probation of Offenders Act in 1907 the state assumed certain responsibility for social welfare work. The consent of the offender was required before he could be put on probation and this is still the case today. Any break in probation regulations could bring him back to the court. The act stated that the character, antecedents, age, health, and mental condition of the offender; the trivial nature of the offense; and extenuating circumstances were to be taken into account by the courts when making the probation order. The probation officer was required to "advise and befriend." The act was the first step toward an official salaried service of social workers attached to the courts.

Other statutory services were improving the material condition of the poor, but the task of helping probationers to find jobs and homes was still formidable. In those days, from the point of view of treatment, the outstanding features were the official recognition of the value of reformative work and the responsibility placed on the probationer himself to accept and justify the chance given.

Further progress came with the Criminal Justice Act of 1925 and the Criminal Justice (Amendment) Act of 1926 which were wider in scope and deeper in application. They pointed the way toward making use of factors other than material aid. Interest in medical and psychological aspects of crime and social inadequacy was growing fast. The first child guidance clinics and psychiatric departments were now available for diagnosis, and sometimes treatment of special factors, such as mental illness, maladjustment, and mental deficiency. This fostered an emphasis on the importance of personal mental factors in delinquency and its treatment, as opposed to the purely environmental.

The report of the 1927 Departmental Committee on the Treatment of Young Offenders spoke of "the importance of adequate medical and psychological reports on the function of the mind." Hitherto there had been little concern with the possible significance of childhood maladjustments, or family relationships, or with the use of a personal and professional relationship between social worker and client.

Between 1938 and 1947 there was added pressure to improve conditions as evacuation in the war years revealed the conditions of poverty and squalor in which many people lived. The separation of husband from wife and father from children emphasized the importance of human relationships, and it became more apparent where good social work could help.

The 1948 Criminal Justice Act, which repealed and replaced the Probation of Offenders Act, 1907, included in its new provisions one which sanctioned and regulated the making of conditions for mental treatment. It recognized that some offenders, while not certifiably insane or defective, and not legally irresponsible, are still so emotionally or mentally unstable that without psychiatric treatment they are unlikely to behave in a manner that would keep them from reappearing in court.

In accepting the need for this provision, however, the act made stringent safeguards against its misuse. Before such an order can be made, a report is required from a doctor "experienced in the diagnosis of mental disorders" stating that the offender both needs and might respond to mental treatment. The probationer still has his right to accept or refuse the condition. It may be added that, while a client is undergoing institutional treatment, the probation officer is relieved of his supervisory function, but not of his duty to "befriend."

The probation officer is conscious that he is dealing with an individual in a particular place and environment. He has contact with the police, but is advised not to become too clearly identified with them. He also has contact with parents who need help and with families in distress. His links with the child guidance clinic, adult psychiatric service, headmasters and school welfare services, health visitors, doctors, and almoners can all help him with his probationers. The school welfare service and headmasters' reports can be of vital importance if the delinquency of a dull child might be attributed to extreme backwardness and lack of satisfying achievement at school. The child's outlook might be changed completely by admission to a special school. The advice of doctors and health visitors may help considerably where matrimonial or delinquency problems are linked with ill health or physical disability.

Against this background of national progress Aberdeen City was developing its probation service. In 1841 Sheriff Watson of Aberdeen and a few other citizens opened an industrial school for boys. With the help of the police, juvenile mendicants were apprehended under an old police act and brought to the school where they were fed and given some education and work and returned to their own homes at night.

The Industrial School Association also made use of the Reformatory School Act of 1854 which authorized the police "to apprehend every young person found begging or wandering, without having any settled place of abode or proper guardianship, and take him before the magistrate." After intimation to the parent, the young person could be transmitted to an industrial school "there to be detained until he be fifteen years of age or legally discharged."

It was not until 1931 that the Aberdeen Town Council appointed its first part-time probation officer. The department now has nine full-time officers, including two women. Each probation officer has about 50 cases. The courts make considerable use of the probation service, which is housed in the same building as the juvenile court, contributing to practical and easy cooperation.

The probation service in Scotland is administered by the Secretary of State whose authority functions through the Scottish Home and Health Department. Each probation area (a county or large burgh or a combination of such areas) has a probation committee. The Sheriff, with any sheriff-substitute whom he may nominate and any stipendiary magistrate exercising jurisdiction within the area, are ex officio members. The remainder of the committee are lay people appointed by the local authority.

The three main duties of the probation committee are to appoint probation officers, to supervise their work, and to ensure that the service is paid for. It is the duty of the local authority to appoint members of the probation committee, the clerk and other officials (other than probation officers), and to supply funds.

During 1962, in Aberdeen, 219 children and young persons (under 17) and adults, were placed on probation for periods of one to three years. The Aberdeen Probation Committee uses a justice of the peace court under Section 50 of the 1937 act, instead of a formal magistrates' court for juvenile offenders as is the case in the other three Scottish cities. The justice of the peace court, with its "sitting" chairman (one has recently retired after occupying this voluntary position for 26 years), and two justices of the peace, one of whom must be a woman, is a much more workable and progressive background in which to deal with young offenders, than is the case in the other cities, where different magistrates preside every week, destroying any continuity of personality or policy.

Approved Schools

An "approved" school is an institution designated by the Secretary of State for Scotland for the purposes of the Children and Young Persons (Scotland) Act, 1932. This act made provisions for the detention and care of children between the ages of 8 and 17 who are committed by the courts for offenses against the law. Such schools in Scotland are managed by a board which is responsible to the Secretary of State. Well over 90 per cent of pupils in approved schools in Scotland have appeared in court on a charge involving theft or burglary. The remainder have faced a wide variety of charges including breach of probation bond, vagrancy, malicious mischief, and occasionally more serious offenses. About 65 per cent of the offenders committed to approved schools have made at least two earlier court appearances.

Approved schools are not equipped to deal with children who suffer from serious mental abnormalities or certifiable mental defects. However, a large number of the pupils are of poor ability and intelligence quotients of less than 85 are very common.

Children committed by the courts to approved schools can be classified as follows:

1. Offenders—children over the age of eight who have been found guilty of an offense punishable, in the case of an adult, with imprisonment. A child under eight years of age cannot be found guilty of an offense.
2. Truants—children of school age who, without adequate reason, have failed to attend an ordinary school regularly and, in the opinion of the court, must be sent to an approved school to ensure that they receive adequate education.
3. Children in need of care and protection.
4. Refractory children, that is, those beyond the control of their parents.
5. Children under 17 under the supervision of a probation officer and shown by him to the satisfaction of the court to need approved school training.
6. Children under the care of a local authority who need the training of an approved school in their own interests.

Aberdeen's old Industrial School has now been replaced by Oakbank Approved School which houses an average of 130 boys at a time between the ages of 13 and 15 years. The school is used to treat the more difficult juvenile offenders. There is firm discipline but much recreational and social activity is provided. Vocational training includes a large market garden and workshops for plumbing, joinery, painting, and cobbling. These are in addition to general school studies and religious instruction. The school has eight full-time teachers and other staff.

The headmaster stresses the need for close liaison between the school and the psychiatric services. Each boy is interviewed by a psychologist within his first month, but after he has had a chance to lose his early hostility. If psychologist and teachers deem it advisable, the boy is then examined by a psychiatrist, and it can follow that he becomes a psychiatric inpatient or outpatient.

Local girls are usually sent to approved schools in Edinburgh, but two voluntary associations also help young girls who are near-delinquents. These are King Street Home and the St. Clair's Home for Girls, which take girls from age 14 to about 19. Girls may come straight from prison, or be recommended to the superintendent by parents, guardians, clergy, doctors, etc. They may be sent from other training homes or they may be nondelinquent migrants who arrive in Aberdeen destitute. An attempt is always made to find employment for them.

Role of Voluntary Agencies

Many of the 40 or so voluntary societies and institutions in the city of Aberdeen were founded in the nineteenth century. Among the earliest were the Sick Man's Friendly Society founded over 160 years ago, the Aberdeen Public Soup Kitchen, and the Rent Aid Association, all of which are still carrying on their work.

The Aberdeen Association for Improving the Conditions of the Poor, which was started in 1870 and at that time was concerned almost entirely with giving material relief, is now one of the largest comprehensive social service agencies in the country. The story of its development is an excellent record of the growth of social thought and action in the region. Even in the very early days there was a pioneering spirit which would do credit to any modern agency. An example was the day nursery which the association started in 1871 to care for children whose mothers went to work.

The nursery cost about threepence a child per day for care from 5:30 A.M. to 6:30 P.M., including food. Another early pioneering effort was the association's employment register of 1871 which aimed to bring the unemployed and prospective employers together.

ABERDEEN ASSOCIATION OF SOCIAL SERVICE. After the Second World War rapid changes took place. The association appointed its first professional caseworker in 1946. Almost as important because of the advanced view it underlined was the alteration of the name to "Aberdeen Association of Social Service" in the following year. At the same time, training of social work students was started, and has since expanded so that the association now takes students from all parts of Britain for field training.

In 1948 the association launched a family holiday scheme. In 1963, 80 children and 67 adults were sent on holiday. Holidays are arranged for mothers who are tired and harassed. They may be sent on their own, and other arrangements made for their children, such as a week or two at the Children's Shelter, a small home run by the association. Holidays may be useful in assisting individuals and families to cope with crises such as bereavement. The flexibility of the voluntary organization is evident in this form of service. When a special case arises, such as an elderly woman who does not want a holiday in the countryside around Aberdeen, but who wants to visit a married daughter or son living in the south of England, the holiday fund can be used to pay for such traveling expenses and a little pocket money.

In the years from 1951 to 1962 one important project undertaken by the Association of Social Service was a working party to study the problem of the "persistent offender." Since the early days the work of the local Discharged Prisoners' Aid Society has been one of its functions. It is the only one of these societies in Scotland to have the services of a professional caseworker.

The Association of Social Service now has five professional family caseworkers and a child care officer. Casework is carried out in close association with other voluntary agencies throughout the city, such as statutory and voluntary children's homes, the Citizens' Advice

Bureau, the City and County Society for the Prevention of Cruelty to Children, the Old People's Welfare Council, the Mother and Baby Home, the Committee for the Welfare of the Disabled, and the Marriage Guidance Council.

Before the last war, homeless unmarried mothers were usually admitted to St. Clair's Home for Girls. During the war a small independent committee developed the Aberdeen Mother and Baby Home. Its object is "to care for and instruct unmarried mothers who for any reason cannot be looked after by their own relatives, and to give their babies as good a start in life as possible." A caseworker from the Association of Social Service is available to the Home, and while advice as to the future of both mother and baby is always given, it is stressed that the mother herself makes the decision whether or not to have the baby adopted. It is now 21 years old and has cared for 1116 girls and 1020 babies. In 1963, 84 girls were admitted and 31 male and 30 female babies were born. Of these, 16 babies went home with their mothers, 4 to domestic posts with mother, 16 were adopted, 6 went straight from hospital to other accommodation, 11 were taken into the care of the Children's Department, 1 died in hospital, and 7 were still in residence at the end of the year.

MENTAL HEALTH ASSOCIATION. In 1951 the association launched the Aberdeen and North-East Association for Mental Health. This body, whose executive committee includes both professional psychiatric workers and lay people, aims to foster interest in the principles of mental health by such means as public lectures, publications and representation to statutory bodies; to create interest in such major social problems as the backward, the delinquent and the mentally handicapped; to participate in the after-care of those recovering from nervous and mental illness, and to give support to the provision of therapeutic social activities, such as clubs and recreational centers. It is in the field of after-care that some of its most significant work has been done so far. It is negotiating the setting up of a day center for mentally handicapped children. This will be professionally staffed and will be for children under five years of age, and ineducables between five and sixteen.

OLD PEOPLE's WELFARE COUNCIL. Since its inception in 1945 the Aberdeen Old People's Welfare Council has established and maintains six homes, all with single or double rooms; six day clubs for old people, three of which provide a chiropody service; a lunch club where meals cost about 1/– (approximately 14 cents) a panel of home visitors and a lodgings scheme. The latter aims to keep old folk in the environment they know best and in which they are most secure. It also contributes toward the cost of a caseworker for old people. This voluntary council was well ahead of the local government in providing old people's homes. The policy was first to build and then ask the public for money, the initial interest-free loan coming from the Association of Social Service.

MARRIAGE GUIDANCE COUNCIL. The Marriage Guidance Council was started in Aberdeen in 1948. During 1963, 70 cases were opened and 55 closed, of which 14 gave indication of improvement. The counsellors are all voluntary and undergo severe assessment and thorough training before being allowed to counsel. They can have immediate advice from the Association of Social Service family caseworkers, and other specialists such as psychiatrists, ministers, and lawyers.

COMMITTEE FOR THE WELFARE OF THE DISABLED. This committee links the work of various local societies for handicapped people. These include the British Diabetic Association, the British Limbless Ex-servicemen's Association, Multiple Sclerosis Society, the Society for Mentally Handicapped Children, Aberdeen Town and County Association for Teaching the Blind in their Homes, Aberdeen and North-East Society for the Deaf, the British Polio Fellowship, Aberdeen and District Spastics Association, and the Rheumatism and Arthritis Association. As a link between these agencies, it helps to prevent overlapping. Statutory bodies such as the Health and Welfare Department, the Education Committee, and the Probation Department are also represented.

LINN MOOR HOME FOR CHILDREN. Linn Moor has for many years been a local home for children in the now obsolete "fresh air fortnight" tradition when, in the days of highly prevalent tuberculosis, children in need of rest, nutrition, and convalescence were sent for a holiday or for recuperation. In the autumn of 1963 Linn Moor reopened as Scotland's one and only residential home for trainable but ineducable mentally handicapped children.

CONCLUSION. The needs for voluntary bodies in the welfare society are those created by the gaps not yet closed by statutory service. This selective review demonstrates that such gaps are real, and that the philanthropic resources are still ready to meet them. Moreover, expansion rather than contraction has been a constant theme since their inception, despite the advent of state organized welfare. Indeed, the appearance of new government social service may, by its very circumscription, highlight unmet needs. Where a continuing demand is clear, as with financial distress, a statutory service may eventually take over the work of voluntary societies, but in these cases the pattern has been their adaptation to other needs rather than dissolution. In this way hitherto unperceived problems are uncovered and higher levels of welfare achieved.

The central feature of the role of voluntary agencies in the welfare society is that, far from being in competition with the state service, their complementarity leads to cooperative integration. While maximum effectiveness through functional coordination has yet to be reached, their role is so assured that total social welfare as we understand it could not be secured in their absence.

REFERENCES
1. Greenland, C. One hundred years of Scottish lunacy legislation: A critical review. *Public Health* 62:147–155, 1958.

2. Henderson, D. K. *The Evolution of Psychiatry in Scotland.* Edinburgh: E. & S. Livingstone, Ltd., 1964.
3. Hunter, R., and Macalpine, I. *Three Hundred Years of Psychiatry, 1535–1860.* London: Oxford University Press, 1963.
4. King, J. (Ed.) *The Probation Service.* London: Butterworth and Co., Ltd., 1958.

Recruitment and Training
for Mental Health

Successful recruitment to mental health services depends upon a number of factors. First, there is the general awareness of the problem by the community at large and, in particular, by groups of key people who play a crucial part in determining public attitudes and action. These include people responsible for determining public policies and the administration of the health services, teachers, members of the medical profession, and parents. Public attitudes are also determined by the mass communication media, such as radio, television, and the press.

In a comparatively small, closely knit, and stable community, such as the northeast region, clearly the "corporate spirit" is of crucial importance—the way in which a series of individual actions combine to give a general impression for or against particular types of social action. It is true to say that at times public opinion in the region has been critical or even hostile to mental health goals but for the most part there has been a growing awareness and a most encouraging increase in the total effort, both official and voluntary, that has gone into solving many of our problems.

The second factor is the status of the psychiatrist, the nurse, and other mental health workers within the community. This has not always been particularly high, partly because recruitment has been inadequate in numbers and quality and partly because it is only recently that the public has been made aware of the very real achievements in mental health. Much of the stigma of mental illness, for instance, has undoubtedly been due to ignorance about the chances of improvement or recovery from serious mental illness, which compare favorably with the chances of recovery from any other group of diseases. The tendency on the part of psychiatrists and nurses to keep themselves apart, shut in behind the walls of the mental hospital, also prevented the public from finding out what was being done. The surrounding mystique was clearly bad for psychiatry, but efforts to open up mental hospitals for psychiatrists, nurses, and others to give talks on their work and to contribute to the local press have helped to break down barriers.

A third factor is the training opportunities for doctors, nurses and others. The northeast has been well placed in this respect since the university medical school is at the focal point of the whole service and can therefore exercise considerable influence on the pattern of recruitment and training. Mental hospitals have been recognized as training schools for nurses for many years and there has been comparatively little difficulty until recently in attracting young men and women to the nursing profession. Opportunities are determined by the quality of training facilities offered. Much still remains to be done since the physical conditions under which doctors and nurses must work and patients must be treated are still far from satisfactory. It is the contrast between the grim appearance of the mental hospital and the glamorous image of the general hospital that makes it more difficult to attract the average person to mental health work. However, recent experience with an entirely new unit in a new building, the Ross Clinic, has shown that interest can be aroused simply by having facilities and living and working conditions which compare favorably with general hospitals.

On the whole, recruitment to all branches of the mental health service has been improving steadily, but quite severe logistic problems remain and might increase in the future as a real manpower shortage at this level of skill and intelligence becomes manifest. The problem is that of increasing the efficiency of the individual worker, because it is certain that as demand increases a further increase in numbers cannot be expected automatically.

Staffing Structure in the Mental Health Service

MEDICAL STAFFING. Medical staff in mental health formerly consisted of a small number of psychiatrists concentrated within the mental hospital with clinical and administrative authority vested in the statutory position of physician superintendent. Thus a rigid, hierarchical structure existed that served its purposes well until psychiatry became a more successful specialty, extended its field of interest to outpatient departments and community care, and a larger proportion of senior men were recruited.

Since salary scales are identical in psychiatry as in other parts of the hospital service, it was logical to expect that the staffing structure might also be uniform (Table III). The recommendations of the Platt Report on staffing structure in the hospital service in Britain has borne out this expectation. It is now clear that the mental health service should be organized on the assumption that the individual consultant psychiatrist is the person primarily responsible for the care and treatment of the patients under his charge. It is recommended that the consultant should work with one or possibly two other colleagues in a "firm" with appropriate supporting staff, which would consist of a permanent junior grade of medical assistant and of recent graduates holding training appointments as house officers or registrars.

An important feature of the Platt Committee's recommendations is that the training grade of senior registrar should be established independently of service needs, so that they would not be expected to play an indispensable part in the running of the service. They would be appointed some four years after graduation for a period of four or five years, during which time they would be given all the facilities for systematic clinical and research training and for secondment to other departments and centers in the region, in other regions, and abroad. Since psychiatry is still an underdeveloped subject and since the training opportunities for senior registrars will in the future be extremely attractive, it is likely that there will

TABLE III. *Staffing structure in the National Health Service, 1963*

Seniority	Grade	Years post-graduate	Duration of appointment	Training
Junior Staff {	House Officer	1	6 months	Yes
	Senior House Officer	2	6–12 months	Yes
	Junior Hospital Medical Officer	3–4	Permanent	No
	Registrar	3–4	2 years	Yes
Senior Staff {	Senior Registrar	4–9	4 years	Yes
	Senior Hospital Medical Officer	Indefinite	Permanent	No
	Consultant	Indefinite	Permanent	No

be enhanced recruitment to psychiatry as a result of this enlightened scheme.

The "firm" system for consultants and supporting staff allows much greater flexibility so that individual firms can take on their clinical responsibility for patients from the time they are seen in their homes or in outpatient departments right on through inpatient treatment and follow-up. Thus continuity of care is much more easily achieved.

UNDERGRADUATE EDUCATION. Most bright medical students have probably narrowed their choice of career to one or two possibilities some time before they graduate. This may be because they have come in contact with the subject that attracts them and possibly also with teachers whose approach and personality appeals to them. It is natural that first choices will more often be made in relation to internal medicine or surgery where first-class teachers and clinicians are never in short supply and where there has been long-term contact between teacher and student. It is a somewhat different matter in psychiatry where there are still comparatively few full-time teachers in Britain and their contact with students is on the whole much less intensive than in other major clinical subjects. However, in Aberdeen, the university department has gradually increased in numbers and in its clinical contact with students. This has resulted in an encouraging degree of interest among senior students and young graduates in taking up psychiatry as a specialty, or at least in spending some time within it before taking up general practice or some other field.

The main undergraduate teaching is a five-week attachment scheme at the Ross Clinic. The student comes in contact with early, mild, and common disorders where active physical, psychological, and social programs are in operation and where response to treatment can be shown in a reasonable time. Since the clinic has close links with the general practitioner and the local authority services, it is possible for him to see clinical problems in proper perspective. There are also opportunities for a few to take posts as clinical clerks in the two mental hospitals. These provide a first-hand knowledge of the working of the hospitals and in many cases have proved to be the crucial experience in the student's decision to take up psychiatry as a career. Another more recent stimulus has been the financing of students to carry out supervised research during vacations.

There is an inherent attraction in the subject for able, mature, and imaginative people. In the past they may often have been put off by the very poor facilities and career prospects. More are now seeing the future as promising and the chance to contribute to the raising of standards as a real challenge. There have always been the less competent and less stable individuals who have looked to psychiatry either as a soft option or as an area where they can work out their own personal problems. Keener competition for vacancies at all levels has made it less possible for them to find a niche in this specialty.

POSTGRADUATE EDUCATION. Postgraduate education is largely based on the apprenticeship principle. It is provided by rotation of staff at registrar and senior registrar levels through the various units in the integrated service. Thus an individual psychiatrist-in-training works in the two larger mental hospitals and the Ross Clinic, and has experience of outpatient work with both adults and children. Arrangements are made with the two mental deficiency hospitals for temporary attachments of junior staff for training. Special interests, for instance in delinquency or in forensic psychiatry, can be catered to by giving senior registrars appropriate experience in the two prisons, the local approved school, and the courts. Similarly, special experience in research, psychosomatic medicine, or child psychiatry can be offered.

In addition to clinical training under supervision, formal courses in psychology, physiology, and general psychiatry are organized for those studying for their Diploma in Psychological Medicine. There is supervised instruction in individual and group psychotherapy. Weekly seminars and other academic activities are supplemented from time to time by symposia organized by the university department. Facilities for individual study are also provided by the department of anatomy and in several general wards of the Royal Infirmary. All psychiatric training, though largely initiated by the university department, takes place entirely within the health service units where there is an abundance of case material available and where the trainee has to rely heavily upon the training skills of the senior clinicians and others with whom he works.

The opportunities for postgraduate training are likely to improve with the new arrangement for training senior registrars. Already, plans are advanced for a year's course in psychotherapy which will be offered to all senior registrars, including some from other regions. More systematic opportunities will be offered for clinical, laboratory, and social research projects under supervision, allowing the senior registrar to take a higher degree. There will also be more intensive courses of study in general medicine, leading to Membership of the Royal College of Physicians. It is unlikely that there will be any restriction on the number of senior registrars, except by the available training facilities, because recruitment to consultant level in psychiatry is still far short of target and likely to be so for many years.

NURSING. There has been a long and honorable tradition of mental nursing in northeast Scotland. Recruits have come mainly from the farming and fishing districts but also from Aberdeen itself. There is now a fairly serious recruitment problem brought about by the creation of new posts in hospitals and the community, and also by keener competition from other nursing fields, the social services, business, and industry. Greater efforts have been needed to modernize and improve training to attract a wide spectrum of recruits for all levels of nursing skills.

Training for mental nurses is mainly organized by the Royal College of Nursing. In-service training for state registered nurses lasts three years. Student nurse salaries are competitive and attractive—indeed better than for general nursing. The two larger regional mental hospitals are recognized training centers. As in general training, systematic instruction is based on the "block" system with practical training on wards. Student nurses are withdrawn for periods from ward training in groups or "blocks" and given class-room instruction. The two hospitals are now combining in a group scheme which will include training in mental deficiency, and there is also much closer contact with the general nurse training schools. This movement will not only result in more varied training for the mental nurse, but will also allow general nurses to spend some eight weeks in practical mental health instruction. The double training will then last five years or less instead of the present six.

One important feature in the new scheme is the greater emphasis on experience in outpatient work and in community care. There is little doubt that the mental nurse of the future will have much more active contact with psychiatrists and social workers in the community. One contribution, resulting from the emergence of the concept of the therapeutic community, relates to group treatment as described on pages 609–610.

Some headway is being made in exploring the possibility of using the mental nurse in community care. For many years psychiatrists have taken an active part in the domiciliary consultation service. More recently, in collaboration with the general practitioners, domiciliary treatment has been attempted in certain groups of patients. Here the mental nurse can work with the consultant. An additional role that has been considered is for mental nurses to take a more active part in follow-up with patients who have been under their care in the mental hospital. Since they are likely to have had a closer relationship with these patients than anyone else in the service, it seems logical that they should be able to maintain relationships after patients are discharged.

THE HEALTH VISITOR.   Health visitors are trained in general and maternity nursing together with an additional year in health education and prevention. The health visitor is the key nurse in the local authority service and will increasingly play a crucial part in local health authority community mental health services. Special courses in mental health have been initiated in Glasgow for some health visitors, enabling them to act as liaison officers between the hospitals and the local authority. Many are attached to mental hospitals and work in the closest collaboration with hospital psychiatrists and psychiatric social workers.

Recruitment and Training of
Other Mental Health Workers

Psychiatric social workers, educational psychologists, probation officers, and child welfare officers all have their own training programs, organized mainly on a national level. There is an overall shortage of social workers of all types in the country and in the region. It is difficult to know how best to attract more workers into these fields. The most promising step is for each region to set up its own more intensive training program. It is likely that in the next few years the new university department of social science will take over training for social work in close association with the local authority and various social agencies. This may assure a steady flow of new recruits into the regional service.

Recruitment and Training of
Voluntary Workers

Voluntary work in mental health is hampered partly by the inherent complexity and mystery of mental illness in the eyes of laymen and partly because there are few clear-cut voluntary activities comparable to those that have proved of so much worth in other fields. For instance, most mental patients are not physically ill or frail and do not require amenities appreciated by the bedridden. Perhaps the major problem is that of communication between so-called normal people and the mentally ill. Impairment of verbal and non-verbal communication in a sick individual makes communication exceedingly distressing for those close to him; for comparative strangers, communication can be simply bewildering.

In the northeast region it has been felt that perhaps the most effective way to encourage voluntary work is to offer special training for those who wish it. Some years ago the Mental Health Association organized training courses from which grew the organization later to be known as "The Friends of Kingseat and the Royal Mental Hospital." This body is now very large indeed but has its core of relatively informed laymen who have been able to give it proper direction.

Both the Marriage Guidance Council and the Aberdeen Telephone Samaritans have relied upon professional workers for instruction in mental health and illness, leading to a very close functional relationship between them and the mental health service (see page 589). The university department has for many years offered instruction in mental health to divinity students as part of their course in practical theology, again resulting in close working relationships with clergymen in the region. Additional courses have been arranged *ad hoc* from time to time for interested clergymen.

CONCLUSION

The fact that there are now so many more active workers in the field has in itself brought the problem of mental health to public notice. Voluntary workers talk much more freely among their friends and many contribute to the mass media. Relatives and patients are now much less afraid of the stigma of mental illness and are able to talk about it more openly and with greater understanding and tolerance. But perhaps the most important aspect of the training and recruitment drive in the region has been that it has brought so many varied types of individuals into close functional and personal contact with one another. Patients, relatives, friends, voluntary workers, and professionals are all being welded into a community dedicated to mental health goals.

THE INTEGRATED
REGIONAL MENTAL
HEALTH SERVICE

Introduction

So far the aim has been to show how various social, philosophical, administrative, legal, and medical influences have contributed to the development of an integrated social and mental welfare system in Britain and how this national movement has found expression in the specific locality of northeast Scotland. The second part of this book is devoted to a detailed exposition of some of the more salient aspects of mental health services in relation to total social welfare. A corollary of integrated social welfare is an integrated system of community mental health services in which the role of psychiatry becomes defined, not merely as a branch of medicine, but ultimately as a network of relationships touching every aspect of welfare.

The import of this philosophy is that mental welfare, as part of total social welfare, must be seen to be in and of the community, rather than imposed from outside; as part of infrastructure rather than superstructure. In this sense integration becomes a cooperative system of flexible links effecting rational administration and organization in continuous compromise with the infinitely changing variety of community and individual needs. It is at the point when services begin to be designed around individual and group needs rather than in terms of some global administrative convenience or moral dogma that community mental health becomes a practical reality. Though the northeast region is far from this ideal, it has already gone some way toward evolving a pattern of services which is truly regional and truly integrated both internally and in relation to community social welfare as a whole.

The processes which bring patients into psychiatric care are not well understood, but at least community-wide facility of access can be ensured. How this is effected in this region is described on pages 577–592. The second chapter in this section recounts the evolution of general hospital psychiatry and its eventual transformation into a regional center which has become the nucleus for a system of regional services (Figure 4, p. 603). The third chapter in this part relates the mental hospitals to the regional complex of services, first as seen from one of the larger mental hospitals, and second from the point of view of a small rural district unit which is rapidly becoming a comprehensive community mental health center in the American sense. The fourth chapter in the section deals with four prominent problems which are common to most psychiatric service systems. Psychogeriatrics, mental deficiency, child psychiatry, and alcoholism are examples of special groups requiring special kinds of service to meet unique needs. The final chapter gives a general account of services designed to rehabilitate the patient and his community, in which mutual adjustment is seen to be central.

It cannot be claimed that the ground has been covered completely, or even adequately. To do so would require several volumes such as this. It is hoped that these glimpses will be enough to stimulate thought, if not provoke controversy.

Paths to
the Psychiatric Services

The popular theme of community psychiatry seems at times to have as many definitions as there are workers in the field. Certainly one cannot describe the various agencies of referral of psychiatric patients without using this concept. The pendulum in psychiatry has swung from the closed to the "open door" policy with all the permissiveness and raising of anxiety that this can produce. The community is morally and legally committed to this way of thinking. In Scotland there has always been a strong social conscience as far as the less fortunate members of our community are concerned. The guardianship system for the care and protection of the mentally handicapped has been in operation for decades. Now, with the "new" Mental Health (Scotland) Act, 1960, increasing emphasis is being placed on the community to take the strain of the problem of mental illness and mental deficiency which traditionally has been hospital-orientated for so many years.

This then is producing a social revolution in thinking about the problem of the mentally ill. Hospitals so long regarded as the "asylum" of the afflicted must be seen by the man in the street as something different. The quickening movement came from within. Hospitals began to think again of social processes, long known but forgotten. There was an upsurge of activity and enthusiasm with the advent of the "open door" policy represented by Bell of Dingleton Hospital, Melrose, and now extended far and wide.

Another concept gradually emerged—the therapeutic community. This is not easy to define; everything that is going on between patient and staff is worthy of discussion and interpretation as a healing situation, surely a challenging proposition. Everyone is affected positively or negatively. No one can remain out of such a process. Difficulties arise in the role of the nurse and doctor and even in the role of the patient. Personal liberty is the order of the day. We have to ask ourselves what is legal, social, or psychiatric liberty. There are members of the medical and nursing profession who cannot accept the changes involved for they are too threatening and the wish at times is for their removal or destruction. There is nothing new in the concept of the therapeutic community. Dickens in his travels in America remarked on the physician superintendent of a mental hospital sitting down with his family to "sup" with the patients.

If the liberalizing movement of the last decade has caused heart-searching in the hospitals and clinics among professional workers in the field, it has also had a continuing effect on the citizens of our communities. There was an element of dread and yet safety in the traditional approach to the mentally ill. They were "put away" with plausible logic: they were sick in a certain way and had to be protected from themselves, and society also must be protected. This attitude is still present today but to a lessening extent and one feels that change in the public attitude alters in direct ratio to the effectiveness and humanity of the psychiatric services offered to the community.

Society must come to terms with present concepts of mental illness. It must be encouraged to accept the hospital setting as only a stage in the reorganization of the individual. Communities must take more responsibility for the sick in mind. It is with these hopes that we concern ourselves with the halfway house, outpatient facilities, the attachment of psychiatric inpatient units to general and other hospitals—all geared to alter the image of the mentally ill person in the eyes of the community.

At the same time we must keep some perspective in this plan. There is no point in inflicting a sick person on a family if by so doing the family is going to be more disintegrated than previously. Yet it is remarkable to note the differences in tolerance levels from family to family and from community to community. Families are known who are coping and willingly so with mentally ill members who would have been extruded long ago by families with lower frustration levels. What decides the level of acceptance? This and similar questions we are only now beginning to tackle.

All this means, in essence, a shift of emphasis from the traditionally hospital-based psychiatric services to the living processes in a community into which we are expecting to inject situations of behavioral abnormality. This will not happen without some reaction; these reactions must be studied. The community must be educated to accept the change and to modify it; the community services for the mentally ill must be increased and supported accordingly. We must use the situation as a learning process to find out what constitutes a mental illness, what decides community tolerance. We must learn to test out our hypotheses on psychiatric illness in the context of the interaction between man and man and not in the back ward of a mental hospital.

There are many ways members of the community can come into contact with the psychiatric services in the northeast of Scotland. These are shown in detail in Figure 3, and it can be seen that there are a number of overlapping situations which can occur in patient referral. This is advantageous because it allows the collection of various aspects of the potential patient's problems. In addition, the northeast is small enough to allow the maximum interdepartmental and inter-staff contact—most valuable assets in a psychiatric setting. One criticism of this "closeness" of departments is that on occasions there may be too many people involved in the assessment of a particular problem. However, this is outweighed by the gathering of various skills to the crisis and to its solution on a community basis.

The broad canvas can be shown best by concentrating on the three areas of activity in the National Health Service.

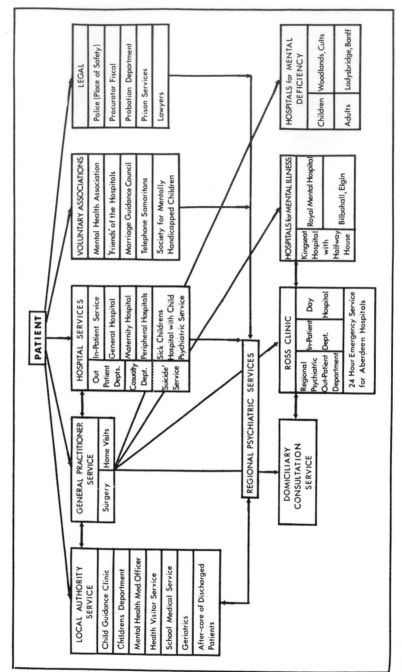

FIGURE 3. *Referral sources, northeast Scotland mental health services.*

GENERAL PRACTITIONER SERVICE

There are 90 general practitioners in the city of Aberdeen itself, and 159 in the mainland counties of the region. Over 97 per cent of the population are registered with a family doctor. Consequently, the majority of patients becoming known to the psychiatric services in the northeastern region do so by initial referral from their particular family doctor. Indeed, this is as it should be because in this country the general practitioner is the backbone of the health services and plays a vital role in keeping the personal link between his patient and himself in contrast to the more remote world of the specialist services and the hospital.

Some patients prefer at the outset to refer themselves and do not want any information on their illness or problem transmitted to the doctor, though it is interesting that those few who initially may have this idea change their minds as a rule when they enter the treatment situation and realize the importance and advantage to themselves of having their general practitioner in the picture. It may be that the patient feels that his particular doctor does not "understand" mental problems; he may feel rejected in discussing such things with him. Generally this can be worked through and seen in the light of problems with authority figures.

The family doctor, having made the decision that a particular patient should be referred, has a number of methods available to him. In the first instance, he can write a summary of the problem and send it to the regional psychiatric outpatient clinic centered on the Ross Clinic. Either this referral can be directed to the appointments clerk or the letter can be addressed to a particular consultant of the practitioner's choice. This allows the doctor to continue to build up relationships with psychiatrists because it is easier for him to talk to someone he knows. This is one of the advantages of working in an area which is small enough to allow general practitioners and hospital staff to be on close terms with one another, often at friendship and first-name level.

If the general practitioner decides that the patient on whom he wishes a psychiatric opinion is not able to go to the psychiatric outpatient clinic, he can elect to have a domiciliary visit carried out by the consultant psychiatrist of his choice. This service has been made use of in the northeast for many years. Not only is it of value to the family doctor who has the initial responsibility of deciding whether the clinical situation is a psychiatric one, it is also of considerable value to the psychiatrist who may be asked to see and probably undertake treatment of the patient. The psychiatry of the home visit is different from the psychiatry of the outpatient clinic and is different again from the situation in the hospital. All manner of important clues are picked up by the trained observer in the domestic scene that may never emerge in the sterility and artificiality of the interviewing room. In addition a ten-minute briefing from the doctor may be worth more than an hour with the patient as the family dynamics unfold and the presenting clinical problem begins to make more sense.

There are other avenues of action for the family doctor. He may feel in the first instance that the clinical situation can be dealt with by calling in the services of the local authority in the form of the health visitor in the district or health visitors specially trained in the problems of mental health. Such officers are known as "mental after-care officers" in terms of the Mental Health Act. In the city of Aberdeen there are two practices to which a health visitor is permanently attached. These practices have the advantage of a known team member being involved in any family situation where mental illness occurs.

Of course, the difficulty in any family situation may not be that of a definitive mental illness such as is generally recognized in psychiatric circles but may be a predominantly social problem, or a school situation or symptoms suggesting the need for a child psychiatrist. Accordingly, the practitioner can refer to the appropriate agency of the local authority or hospital service. For example, he may wish to refer his young patient to the consultant child psychiatrist at the Sick Children's Hospital; or an elderly patient to the local authority "old folks" service, the hospital-based geriatric service, the psychiatric service, or to all three in turn. There is considerable overlapping between these services and at least one member at a clinical level in each has an honorary appointment in the services belonging to the other divisions of the Health Service.

Finally, in psychiatry as in any other branch of medicine, the services of the region are such that if a practitioner wishes to admit a patient directly to a mental hospital he has only to contact the hospital and arrange admission.

Thus the method of presentation to the psychiatric service is fluid and non-rigid.

Many practitioners are far from content to admit a patient to the psychiatric services as either an outpatient or inpatient and let the service deal with the problem. His experience in practice has led him to accept the far-reaching implications of mental disturbance in any family setting and it is vital that he be kept informed as to what is happening to his patient. This means writing to him at intervals concerning drug therapy and psychotherapy. Frequently, a telephone call to the doctor is worth more than any letter and keeps the two-way channel of communication going.

A number of doctors are becoming more and more interested in their role as "therapeutic agents" in the psychotherapeutic sense and periodic contact is made with interested practitioners to let them see the dynamics of a particular clinical problem as well as to give the traditional case conference report.

Bound up with the use of a psychiatric service is the doctor's education in the subject of psychiatry. Psychiatry is a difficult subject to teach and it can only have an influence on the future general practitioner if it is well and sensibly taught. The doctor will be much more inclined to refer a patient to a psychiatric setting if he himself is familiar with it. Communication between psychiatrist and doctor is still not of the best. Too few practitioners are seen in the wards of the psychiatric clinic or hospital compared with the wards of a general hospital.

LOCAL AUTHORITY SERVICES

If the general practitioner is seen as the first line of defense in dealing with the mental health difficulties of his patients, then the local authority services must be seen as the lines of communication, support, and reinforcement behind the trenches. This has been recognized for many years and gradually the areas of suspicion between one branch of the National Health Service and the others are being broken down. Cooperation between the three divisions of the service is the order of the day and certainly this is so in psychiatry.

A recent report (1) defined the responsibilities of local authorities and made the following important points in their summary of recommendations:

Community care. The object of every local authority must be to expand their mental health services to the point at which no person need be resident in hospital unless he will benefit from or requires hospital care.

Cooperation. Cooperation between the various bodies providing services for persons suffering from mental disorder is essential. Joint committees representing local authorities, hospitals, general practitioners, and voluntary mental health associations should be established to keep under review existing mental health services and plans for future development.

These are some of the recommendations which were crystallized in Part II of the Mental Health (Scotland) Act, 1960, where the general provisions of the local authority services are laid down.

The whole import of the present situation existing between the general practitioner services, the hospital services, and the local authority services is that of increasing and expanding *cooperation*. In the field of the mental health services it is expected that as time passes there will be set up various joint services sharing staff, accommodation, and expenses. An attempt is already being made to set up a joint assessment clinic in the region covering the needs of both mentally handicapped and physically handicapped children. Members of the assessment clinic will include the general practitioner, local authority, and hospital staff, as the needs of the particular child dictate.

The local health authority has various subservices, all of which may have to deal with the problems of patients who are mentally ill. In addition, there are associated services such as the children's department and education department where often contact has to be made with the psychiatric services. The Medical Officer of Health of the local authority is the integrating officer of all the health services. Within this administrative framework are the following services.

School Medical Service

The medical officers of this service carry out periodic examinations of children of school age. Part of this examination should be directed to the ascertainment of any obvious mental health difficulty such as poor performance at school, the presence of problem behavior, or obvious signs of emotional difficulty. It should be recognized that the class teacher is an important member of the health team in drawing the attention of the physician to any signs of unusual behavior she may have noticed. In this regard, the medical officer may refer the child to the family physician or to the appropriate clinic at the hospital or to the education authority child guidance clinic if it is felt that the problem may be one of remedial education. It may be necessary to recommend transfer of the child to special educational facilities if there is any question of mental or physical handicap obstructing normal educational progress.

The Geriatric Services

There is a close link between the geriatric services of the local authority, the geriatric consultants of the hospital service, and clinical psychiatrists with routine cross-referrals.

Health Visitor Service

Health visitors play an important part in the health services of the local authority. In Aberdeen there is an establishment of 73. The duties are many and varied. One important function of the health visitor is to detect early signs of disturbance in the families she visits and if necessary pass on this information to the family doctor and to her superior.

The Aberdeen City local authority has established the post of Senior Assistant Medical Officer, whose duties are "primarily in the organization, control, and administration of the mental health services" of the local authority. This medical officer is in close contact with his colleagues in the hospital service and calls on them for assistance in the examination of patients that are referred to him in reports from local authority personnel. In short, he is very much a coordinating officer of the local authority services. He may draw the family doctor's attention to any sign of abnormality known from the health visitor's contact with the family. More rarely, requests for psychiatric examination may come from the local authority in terms of their port authority responsibility toward seamen.

Child Guidance Clinic

Children are referred to this clinic principally by school teachers and by medical officers of the school medical service. The principal psychologist in charge of the clinic may refer patients to the regional psychiatric services as is considered necessary and visits are paid to the child guidance clinic as requested. There is also a link with the consultant child psychiatrist and his clinic at the Sick Children's Hospital.

Children's Department

It is not infrequent for very disturbed children to be in the care of the children's departments of local authorities. Such children have been referred to the psychiatric services for many years and this trend will continue. All the serious emotional difficulties of the separated and problem family are commonly bound up with children in care and it is hoped that as the child psychiatric services expand there will be even more close links with children's departments.

HOSPITAL SERVICES

It is clear from reference to Figure 3, that the populations of the general and special hospitals, peripheral hospitals, outpatient departments, and the casualty department and attached ward hold a large number of potential patients for the psychiatric services of the region. Patients may be admitted to any hospital or outpatient setting when, in fact, the appropriate referral may have been known to be, or turns out to be, to the mental health service.

Ward Referrals

Referral from the doctor in charge of the patient may be by letter, or by telephone if an urgent psychiatric opinion is requested. A psychiatrist from the Ross Clinic is available throughout the 24-hour period. The duty psychiatrist is generally of registrar or senior registrar grade and deals with any ward or outpatient department referrals that come his way during his duty day where the referring doctor has not specified any particular psychiatrist. Alternatively, referrals can be addressed to a particular consultant psychiatrist who deals with them himself. Domiciliary psychiatry is undertaken by consultant psychiatrists only.

On the average there is at least one referral per day to the clinic for a psychiatric opinion on a patient in one of the wards of the hospitals in the city. In addition there are at least two medical wards where a contact has been built up between their staff and a particular consultant. In the same way there are of course referrals of patients to the child psychiatrist based on the Sick Children's Hospital.

It seems that the nature of the clinical problems referred over the years has altered in a number of ways. There are the classic psychiatric syndromes such as depression, anxiety state, or dissociative problems, and the florid psychotic conditions, but one now sees much more frequently the psychology of physical illness. Here there is no doubting the "organic" nature of the events in the patient's life, but an opinion is being asked on the handling of the physical condition and the psychopathologic situations that such physical diseases produce. To give examples, there is the patient who develops a coronary thrombosis early in life; the patient with Parkinson's disease and the fear of invalidism; and the special disease problems such as the patient with cancer. There is a whole range of clinical entities and personality structures which can be a learning situation to physician, psychiatrist, and student.

Casualty Department and Casualty Ward

The present casualty department and ward is located in the old general hospital building in a central position downtown. All forms of accident cases in industry, on the roads, and in the home are handled in addition to the everyday run of clinical situations presenting at any casualty department. In addition, as far as is possible, all patients who have made an attempt at suicide by taking an overdose of drugs or coal gas, or by any other means, are admitted to the casualty department as soon as they have become known to the family doctor, police, or other source. There is a routine administration which ensures that *all* patients admitted to the casualty department who have made an attempt at suicide by any means are referred to the psychiatric service at the Ross Clinic. Table IV gives figures for a four-month period.

TABLE IV. *Referrals of "attempted suicide" to the Ross Clinic from wards and casualty department, August–November 1963*

Month	Ward	Casualty Dept.†	Total
August	17	25	42
September	8	20	28
October	19	19	38
November	22	21	43

* This does not take into account ward referrals directly to a particular psychiatrist or the small number of patients who may be admitted to other medical wards with a history of taking an overdose of some substance and who are not referred to the psychiatric service.

† The numbers noted as being referred from the casualty department are, with one or two exceptions, patients who have taken an overdose of some substance, either as a piece of manipulative behavior in a crisis situation, or as a serious attempt to take their own life. All are classified as "attempted suicide."

This form of automatic referral to the service allows information to be gathered on the nature of the problem of attempted suicide over a period. There has been a considerable increase in the number of patients referred from the casualty department in the current year who had made an "attempt" by overdose with some substance.

As against 99 patients referred in 1962, the 1963 figure was in excess of 200 patients. The various factors underlying this change are no doubt complex and warrant further study.

VOLUNTARY AGENCIES

Referrals from the Marriage Guidance Council come in several ways. Most commonly, an individual counsellor will write or phone a senior member of the clinic staff and make an appointment. Occasionally the problem is disposed of by discussion of the case at the time of the initial contact. One consultant psychiatrist acts as regular adviser and supervisor to the counsellors, meeting with them each month and taking part in the case conferences. It has been found that most problems can be dealt with by the counsellors themselves with the help they receive in this way. Clergymen and lawyers also participate in this advisory service and may be brought into certain complex cases along with the psychiatrist.

The problems disclosed through this service include a wide variety of sexual disorders and deviations, cruelty, alcoholism, neglect, incompetence due to mental defect, and paranoid reactions. It is not so common for frank psychotic or neurotic reactions to be uncovered. Usually one member of the partnership is disturbed by the behavior of the other to the point that tolerance has reached breaking point. The possibility that a marriage is about to break up is not perceived by the spouses as essentially a medical problem, and an approach to a lawyer is taken to mean a drastic decision to end the marriage. Because the levels of tolerance in some spouses are neurotically low, the problem lies as much with the complainer as with the one complained of. This being so, the strategy of treatment centers round the nature of the relationship since the partnership began. It is found that well-trained counsellors are both skilled and successful in handling these difficult problems in this way.

The more recently established Telephone Samaritans offer a more general and less specialized service to all who are in distress and in particular to those who are desperate to the point of suicide. The small headquarters are open at all times to receive telephone calls from any source. Most inquiries are made during the daytime and are concerned with such personal problems as hire purchase debts and minor personal emergencies. Very few of the clients who approach this service are perceived by the organization as psychiatric and hence referrals are negligible. Nevertheless, there is a similar arrangement made with the Samaritans as with the Marriage Guidance Council whereby a psychiatrist is available for frequent consultations on special problems. Originally it had been thought that a significant number of suicidally-minded persons would contact the service but this has not proved to be the case. Similarly, there are not many whose crises are of such severity that experts of one kind or another are needed.

The Aberdeen Association of Social Service who, with the local Health and Welfare Department, is most knowledgeable about problem families, from time to time refers cases where it is evident that institutional care is required, or where court action is imminent and a psychiatric opinion will be requested. Again, as with the other two services, there is close and regular collaboration between the hospital staff and the association. There are regular meetings with psychiatric social workers from the Health Service at case conferences where clients with a psychiatric history are discussed.

The comparatively small number of cases referred from these three sources is an indication of, first, the effectiveness of these services; second, the close collaboration with the psychiatric services; and, third, the desirability of this kind of organization. It is mutually agreed that a "psychiatric case" is one that is best dealt with primarily by the psychiatric services. If a person exhibiting signs and symptoms of psychiatric disorder is best dealt with by another service, even a voluntary one, it is not regarded as clinically improper that this should be the disposal of choice. Close personal contact among all workers in the field ensures that the most effective use is made of the resources available.

THE LEGAL SYSTEM

Referrals may come from various legal agencies. General practitioners may refer a patient for a psychiatric opinion because of some offense when the question of mental state has been raised by the police or defending lawyer. It is not infrequent for the Procurator Fiscal to ask for an examination of and a report on the mental state of an accused person. The Mental Health (Scotland) Act, 1960, allows the remand of accused persons in prison or their admission to a hospital for the purpose of such examinations. Probation officers in the course of their enquiries may request a psychiatric examination and report. The police, too, in their day-to-day duties may come across people in the city or county in whom they suspect mental illness. They are empowered to take them to the officially designated "Place of Safety" (a locally specified hospital) where a psychiatric examination can be carried out.

In the Aberdeen area there is also a close link between the psychiatric services and the two local prisons, one of which (Peterhead) detains long-term prisoners. A psychiatrist pays regular visits to Peterhead prison and group methods of therapy have been used with disturbed prisoners. A special psychiatric unit is being set up in the prison for cases arising within it.

Part V of the Mental Health Act has greatly increased the possibility of psychiatric cases being referred to the mental health service rather than being dealt with in the penal system. For many patients that formerly would have been given prison sentences the court has made out a "hospital order," committing them to hospital treatment, sometimes with and sometimes without restriction on discharge. Psychotic and psychopathic murderers are now being so committed, provided they have not been found guilty of a capital crime. It seems likely, therefore, that in the future, where an accused person is thought to be suffering from mental disorder, mental defect, or psychopathic state, the court will deal with his case through a hospital order or perhaps through probation with a condition of psychiatric treatment, rather than proceed to sentence. Thus the old arguments as to criminal responsibility and the like that often brought ridicule to psychiatrists taking up sharply opposing (and therefore inconsistent) points of view, which were neither in the interests of justice nor good medical practice, will probably disappear. They will be replaced by detailed and objective reports, couched in neutral and more technical language, submitted in person or in writing, to the court. In this way the expert opinion of the psychiatrist will be made available in the interests of both the accused person and society.

However, if referrals of criminal cases—many of which will require security precautions—are to increase, then special units will have to be set up for this purpose. At a time when mental hospitals are treating patients for short periods and under "open" conditions it would not work satisfactorily to have the disruptive influence of this group of patients mingled with the rest.

CONCLUSION

There are many formal agencies through which contact with the regional psychiatric services can be made. Cooperation between the various agencies and organizations, though already good, can undoubtedly be improved. The patient can only benefit.

It is beyond the scope of this book to discuss the role of informal community agents in helping people in difficulty to cope. The minister, the grocer, the barman, the family friend, and countless others take part in the everyday processes by which the community takes care of its own. Their contribution is perhaps the most significant factor in keeping within manageable proportions the already high referral rate of 5.66 new adult cases per 1000 of the population per year (2).

REFERENCES

1. Department of Health for Scotland, Scottish Health Services Council. *Mental Health Services of Local Health Authorities*. Edinburgh: Her Majesty's Stationery Office, 1961.
2. Innes, G., and Sharp, G. A. A study of psychiatric patients in North-East Scotland. *J. Ment. Sci.* 108:447–457, 1962.

Psychiatry and the General Hospital: Emergence of the Regional Mental Health Center

ORIGINS—THE UNIVERSITY DEPARTMENT

During the 1930's there was a growing interest in Britain in the development of services for the neuroses. The impetus for this came from the discovery during World War I of shell shock, a condition that interested psychiatrists and neurologists alike, and was a blanket term describing most acute psychoneurotic reactions.

T. A. Ross' *The Common Neurosis* made a profound impression upon British medicine and it was Ross himself whose inspiration led to the setting up in Aberdeen of the university department of psychopathology in 1937. Ross had been invited to deliver a short course of lectures to the faculty of medicine the previous year and this prepared the ground for the inauguration of the new department. The medical stimulus in Aberdeen came from Dr. (later Sir) Alexander Anderson, a noted physician whose interest lay in the neurologic and psychosomatic fields.

At that time psychological medicine had become fossilized in the mental hospitals which were largely custodial institutions and did not make much impact upon the general body of medicine, either in practice or in research. Medical psychiatric education was restricted to a few lectures and demonstrations of gross institutionalized psychosis, conditions that had little relevance to the everyday practice of medicine, either in general practice or in teaching hospitals. It was in order to bring psychological medicine more closely in touch with the rest of medicine that the new department was set up and it was logical that its base should be the general hospital.

The first and only holder of the new lectureship was Dr. Douglas MacCalman. The only other member of the department was a psychiatric social worker, Miss Marion Whyte. Between them they developed outpatient services at the general hospital, the Aberdeen Royal Infirmary, and the Sick Children's Hospital. Three beds were allocated in Dr. Anderson's medical ward in the Royal Infirmary, later to be increased to five.

Teaching of undergraduates in those days remained sketchy. A few extra hours of teaching time were allocated to the department and this gave undergraduates a brief introduction to the neuroses and to child psychiatry. But the classes were poorly attended since they were not regarded as part of the normal curriculum, as was the course in mental diseases. Accordingly, the emphasis was still upon the psychoses as they were manifested within the walls of the mental hospitals.

Some further increase in the scope of the department occurred during the Second World War when additional beds were allocated for "war" neuroses occurring in both the civil and military populations in the area. However, there were severe limitations in staff and facilities so that no major advances could occur until after the war was over.

In 1946 the university authorities, partly on the basis of the favorable experience of the small department's work during the previous eight years, partly because of widespread interest in the growth of the mental health services as a result of war experience, and partly because of the recommendations of various government committees, decided to institute a full professorial department of mental health to replace the department of psychopathology. Dr. MacCalman became the first professor in May of that year, and the way was now open for more rapid advances in both the academic and the service aspects of mental health.

Until 1948 the provision of medical and ancillary services to the teaching hospitals was voluntary. Specialists (except those in the local authority hospitals and the mental hospitals) were expected to give their services free, recouping their losses by private practice. With the introduction of full-time clinical appointments by the university medical school, the university came to provide a significant proportion of the free service in teaching hospitals. It was because of this special situation that the newly formed department of mental health found itself in the somewhat unique position of an academic department charged with the responsibility of developing the whole of the outpatient, children's, and general hospital services on behalf of the teaching group.

THE NATIONAL HEALTH SERVICE

There is little doubt that the 1947 National Health Service Act represented by far the most profound influence for the further development of mental health services in Great Britain. In the northeast region the situation was transformed almost overnight; specialists in psychiatry were for the first time regarded as of equal competence and status to physicians, surgeons, and other specialists within the hospital service. Salaries of all medical, and to some extent nursing, staff were doubled or even tripled, and it is probably true to say that from 1948 onward those in academic psychiatry no longer had to fight for a place in the sun, *vis-à-vis* their more privileged and prestigious colleagues.

However, facilities remained far from ideal. A few beds in the Royal Infirmary and the use of the outpatient facilities in the gynecological department twice a week represented the total resources of the new department of mental health. In those early days, conditions of work were chaotic and teaching was a major burden. Patients would arrive in the morning or afternoon without appointments and the three psychiatrists and one psychiatric social worker had to deal with dozens of cases of all types and severity until well into the evening hours. Patients were still extremely reluctant to come to the psychiatrist and general practitioners referred them only for disposal to a mental hospital. Since there was gross over-crowding in the one hospital remaining at the time, the other (Kingseat) having been taken over as a naval hospital throughout the war, there were few voluntary admissions. Most patients were required to be certified and this sometimes took several hours in any particular case.

THE REGIONAL OUTPATIENT CLINIC

In 1949, accommodation became available for a full-time psychi-atric clinic serving the region. This made an enormous difference to the efficiency of the service and allowed an appointment system to be started. It also permitted the organization on a sessional basis of outpatient work by the staff of the two larger regional mental hospitals (Royal and Kingseat). Thus by 1949 a very considerable increase in patient referrals had taken place and by the early 1950's over 1000 new patients were being referred to this clinic annually; whereas, in 1946, 200 or 300 were the average. There were fewer more seriously ill patients requiring referral to hospital and more suffering from neuroses, psychosomatic disorders, and early psychotic conditions who might be treated at home, or as outpatients.

Since this clinic was part of the general outpatients' service for the main teaching hospital, there were close ties particularly with the medical outpatient department and the casualty service. This allowed for cross-referral of patients throughout the outpatient services and brought psychiatry into closer functional relation with the rest of medicine.

During the late 1940's and early 1950's, following its demobiliza-tion as a naval hospital, Kingseat was again being built up under the active leadership of Dr. Adam Milne. Additions to staff took place, particularly at the trainee level. This allowed for a system of rotation of junior staff between the three main units—the university department of mental health, and the Royal and Kingseat Hospitals. It also permitted a much more integrated functioning of the whole service in that many more patients were now being admitted directly to mental hospitals which were gradually being upgraded, better staffed, and giving both patients and relatives much more hope of active treatment and recovery. To bring about closer integration among members of staff, the university conferred honorary academic status on senior members of Kingseat as well as on Royal Mental staff. Likewise, all university staff were accorded honorary status within the hospitals.

DOMICILIARY PSYCHIATRY

Before 1948 it was the custom for consultants in any specialty to be invited to see patients in their own homes at the request of general practitioners. This had been a feature of British medicine much valued by patients and doctors alike. In 1948 the tradition was perpetuated by an arrangement whereby general practitioners could call out consultants for a specified fee, provided it could be shown by the general practitioner that the patient could not attend an outpatient clinic. For psychiatry, the proviso that the patient should be homebound was largely waived and it was sufficient for the general practitioner to say that it was more in the interests of the patient to be seen in his home than that he should be asked to go some distance to hospital or at some inconvenience. In this way any patient in whom it was thought a mental condition was arising which required psychiatric opinion, was as likely to be seen in his home as in a clinic. The two senior members of the department of mental health and one from the Royal Mental Hospital undertook the major part of this service but any consultant could be specially requested to see patients in their homes.

In the early days the principal function of the consultant psychiatrist was to see patients who were about to be admitted to a mental hospital. Usually he had considerable skill, not only in appreciating the situation, but in smoothing the path for admission, so that gradually the vast majority of patients—up to 80 per cent—were admitted on a voluntary basis. Those requiring to be committed were certified immediately, usually by the psychiatrist and the family doctor. Patients who had been certified by two doctors in terms of the old Lunacy Acts of 1857, usually became the responsibility of the local authority health and welfare departments to arrange transport to hospital. The staff of local authorities were extremely skilled in the art of general persuasion and it is a tribute to their tact and experience that very few patients, even those who were a real danger to themselves and others, gave any major difficulty so far as admission was concerned. Indeed, if a patient had become so violently difficult that the police had to be brought in, they usually took the view that if the authorized officers could not succeed, then it was unlikely that they could do any better! Thus it emerged that patients were being seen at a comparatively early stage in their illness and admitted to hospital before any major crisis arose.

This procedure became more and more simple and straightforward so that ultimately most patients were persuaded easily enough to go into the hospital in their own interests, often by general practitioners who were by this time thoroughly familiar with the process.

TEN BEDS IN THE GENERAL HOSPITAL

By 1953 the outpatient and domiciliary aspects of the service based on the department of mental health were operating smoothly and efficiently. At this time the inpatient service was rudimentary but it was ultimately agreed upon that some ten beds should be made available in one of the medical flats in the Royal Infirmary, specifically for psychiatric patients likely to benefit from the type of treatment offered in an open ward in a general hospital with fairly limited day patient and occupational therapy facilities.

Because the orientation of the department was psychodynamic, patients tended to be admitted who would best benefit by fairly intensive forms of individual and group psychotherapy though physical methods of treatment of all kinds were also available, particularly for mild depressions. The inpatient service became extended in two ways: first, a number of patients scattered throughout the wards in the general hospital, under the care of physicians, surgeons, and others, who were also found to have major or minor psychiatric disorders, were treated in conjunction with the appropriate specialist along psychotherapeutic lines. Thus the number of inpatients under active care at any time was usually about 20 throughout the hospital.

Second, a gradually increasing advisory service was being provided by psychiatrists for various other specialists. This consisted mainly of discussions of the psychological handling of patients with various disorders, not necessarily those suffering from any kind of psychiatric disorder. Thus patients in the ante-natal department were often examined and advice given on the psychological and social problems they presented, which arose from such factors as illegitimacy, broken homes, and marital disharmony. Patients with terminal illnesses who were presenting a real problem in nursing management were seen again and again, and appropriate consultations took place with the medical and nursing staff. Often the department was called in simply to deal with rather awkward, complaining, or paranoid patients who were making life difficult for the clinicians and obstructing the course of treatment. The psychodynamics of these various problem cases were discussed and again the overall management was worked out in collaboration. Surgeons would often consult members of staff with regard to preoperative or postoperative care of certain of their patients, perhaps the young or the very old. This type of service was offered not only by the psychiatrists in the unit, but also by members of the nursing staff, the social worker, the psychologist, and the occupational and art therapists, so that a fair proportion of the work of the unit was carried on outside the small ten-bed ward.

The result was that practical help and advice was seen to be available from psychiatrists on matters relevant to day-to-day running of the hospital. Naturally, many patients suffering from incidental psychosis were referred and usually transferred to a mental hospital, but colleagues throughout the hospital much preferred to make use of their psychiatrists as advisers in dealing with their own cases rather than have them there simply to arrange disposal and transfer of difficult problems. While this state of affairs is very familiar to those working in general hospitals in the United States, it is comparatively rare in Britain and certainly at that time—some ten years ago—it was almost unique. There is little doubt that the dynamic orientations of the staff represented the major factor in bringing it about.

A BALANCED SERVICE

Experience during the 1950's paved the way for a balanced service with the general hospital unit and the two major mental hospitals complementing one another in the kind of work they carried out. One point had to be watched with special care. This was the danger of splitting the service between the general hospitals on the one hand and the mental hospitals on the other. This dichotomy had been applied at the very outset when the department of psychopathology was instituted in 1937, and as the various units began to develop their own character it was evident that serious rivalry might stand in the way of further progress. Therefore, whatever future plans were to be made, it was clear that the general hospital unit based within the teaching department should not be of a size, nor dealing with a turnover of patients, that would seriously compete with the two main mental hospitals.

At that time, admissions to Kingseat were approximately 600 in the year and admissions to the Royal Mental Hospital were about 500. Admissions to the small ten-bed unit in the Royal Infirmary were about 100. Nevertheless, it was felt that if good teaching were to be provided for medical students and if a reasonable service were to be offered for cases suffering from milder types of mental disturbance, then about 30 to 40 beds with a turnover of 300 patients per annum should be the aim. A smaller unit was likely to be inefficient. A larger unit might compete with the mental hospitals and in any event might create very real problems within the general hospital complex, from the point of view of both the staff and the general effect of a large number of psychiatric patients in or near other types of patient groups.

It was clearly desirable to plan for a general hospital type of unit that would provide this larger number of beds and continue the out-patient service very much along previous lines with perhaps a certain improvement in facilities rather than staff. It was also felt that a properly planned unit would act as a focus for the domiciliary service and for various academic and clinical interests throughout the region.

THE REGIONAL MENTAL HEALTH CENTER

In 1958 it was finally decided that a building that was about to be completed as a new admission unit for the Royal Mental Hospital and which was situated in its grounds should be re-sited as the regional treatment unit and the base for the professorial teaching unit of the university. Surprisingly little internal adaptation was required to provide 38 inpatient beds, accommodation for some 12 day patients, and extensive accommodation for the outpatient services. This was so in spite of the fact that the original plan was for some 60 beds for male and female patients who would be suffering from much more serious forms of mental disorder and that only a moderate amount of space had been planned for the outpatient service, required mainly for the follow-up of patients who had been in the Royal Mental Hospital alone.

The new unit, named the Ross Clinic, was opened in July 1959, and almost immediately it was apparent that the venture would be a success. One of the great doubts had been that the professorial unit which had formerly been so closely related to the general hospital was now moving out of that ambit and returning to the center of the mental hospital group of services. Many looked upon this as a retrograde step and thought that especially the milder types of neurosis and other types of cases commonly seen in the general hospital would be most reluctant to come to a unit in the grounds of the mental hospital. The fact that the building was new, the equipment and furnishings modern and attractive, and the whole setting in an extremely pleasant parkland, offset this to a very considerable extent. However, the principal reason for the ease of transition from a general to a mental hospital was the imminence of the Mental Health Act.

The change was geographically not so radical as it might appear. The extensive acreage of the Royal Infirmary, Maternity and Sick Children's Hospital site which also accommodates the medical school, is located immediately adjacent to the almost equally extensive Royal Mental Hospital site on the northwest side of the city, lying on a hill overlooking the sea. This remarkable site had been appreciated as a compound for a complex of hospitals as far back as 1900 by one of the great medical visionaries of Aberdeen, Professor Matthew Hay. By planning the various hospitals on the Foresterhill site close to the Royal Mental Hospital, the necessary conditions were laid down for the creation of a balanced, comprehensive hospital service.

All these geographical, legal, and administrative considerations made for the successful emergence of the new unit as the focal point for the Regional Mental Health Service (Figure 4). It also had the advantage of being the main teaching center for medical students and postgraduates. It was now possible, with the very large turnover of patients, to provide more than enough clinical material for the many purposes which were by this time required in a fairly extensive teaching program for undergraduates, at least as compared with other British medical schools.

In the four years of its operation, the clinic has provided a service more or less as predicted. The number of inpatients admitted in any one year is now rather less than 300 and it is noteworthy that, so far as can be seen, no significant reduction in admissions to the two main mental hospitals has resulted. This can be interpreted in a number of ways but the type of patient now being admitted to the Ross Clinic is perhaps the type that had previously been admitted to the smaller unit in the general hospital and possibly also to various medical and other wards in the Royal Infirmary. The Regional Outpatient Service has continued much as before with no very significant increase in the number of new patients referred as compared with the older clinic, despite an increase in the number of staff.

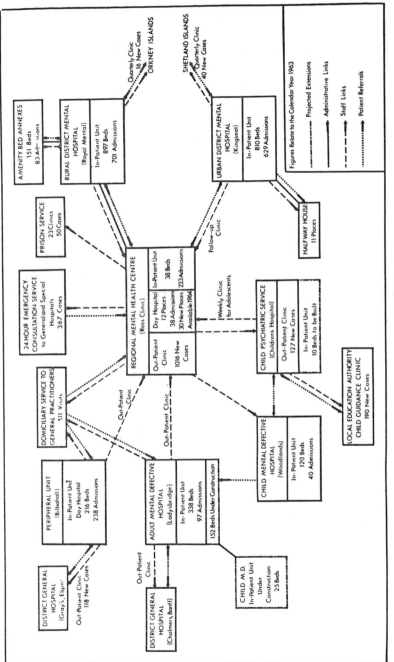

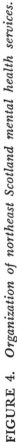

FIGURE 4. *Organization of northeast Scotland mental health services.*

The small, experimental day hospital has functioned in such a way as would indicate that a much more thorough attempt must be made to deal with this whole problem. In 1963, an extension to the clinic was built making provision for some thirty day-patients. This will increase considerably the total volume of work in the clinic. It will also make possible a more significant contribution to the development of a therapeutic community.

CONTINUITY OF CARE

One of the features of a small regional treatment service such as this is that patients are not treated elsewhere than in the regional units. The only private psychiatry in the region is practiced by two National Health Service consultants to the extent of five half-days a week. This means that when patients relapse, they return to the service which cannot escape the responsibility for their continued care and treatment. This forces a certain amount of continuity upon the type of treatment given to patients such that the same patient tends to return sooner or later to the same unit, or even to the same doctor, though "shopping around" does inevitably occur. The need to provide a long-term and comprehensive program of care and treatment for every type of case has forced upon our attention the fact that short bursts of intensive inpatient or out-patient treatment and then discharge in the high hope that the patients will not return is not wise therapeutic planning.

It is equally apparent that much mental disorder is of chronic or recurrent type and that a good service is one that makes best provision for this fact. Accordingly, it has long been felt in this region that different types of facilities, such as outpatient, inpatient, and day-patient care should, if possible, be provided within the same organization, thus enabling any given patient to pass from one facility to another, without complex formality, as the needs of his care demand.

The Ross Clinic consultants who carry out domiciliary visits are also in a position to maintain continuity of care and treatment with outpatients in their own homes. Thus it is possible for any patient at any one time to be under the care of the consultant as an outpatient, as an inpatient, as a day patient, or in his own home, depending on the requirements of his case at the time. Indeed, even greater flexibility can be envisaged in some cases who require spells of inpatient treatment for weekends or even overnight. It is also planned to extend the domiciliary service so that more active treatment can be provided by psychiatrists, social workers, and specially trained nurses. By this arrangement therapy can be "tailor-made" for each patient, depending upon his needs.

Since the Mental Health Act has come into force and the local health authority has begun to play an increasingly important part in the provision of community services, close liaison has been established with local authority health and welfare services. The Ross Clinic, as with Kingseat Hospital, now has local health authority staff attached full-time and working closely with psychiatrists and psychiatric social workers. In this way there is again a smooth transition of care from the hospital to the local authority services with the aim of maximum continuity.

THE ROSS CLINIC PLAN

The Ross Clinic is a comparatively small building subserving several different functions and thereby making the most use of available space. The main part of the building is two-stories and can accommodate 38 inpatients. Most wards have four beds or are single-bed, and one contains eight beds. There is an attractive day room, a fairly large occupational therapy department, and an art therapy department. The rooms mainly occupied by staff comprise for the most part individual consulting rooms, of which there are 16 for medical staff, clinical psychologists, and psychiatric social workers. In the recently opened extension there is a large combined day room and dining room, and a kitchen for day patients and those assigned to group activities. The new records department is also accommodated here. The layout of the ward accommodation is of a size and situation that either male or female patients may occupy any of the single- or four-bed rooms. In this way a high occupancy rate is maintained, despite the fairly rapid turnover. The small wards and single rooms are used in daytime for group therapy and as interview rooms for students. There is a conference room and a small lecture theater in daily use for case demonstrations, staff conferences, and lectures.

One of the agreeable consequences of maximum use of space is that a surprisingly large number of people (patients, staff, students, and visitors) can be accommodated at any one time. Since there is constant movement a high degree of informal communication takes place in the corridors, wards, public rooms, waiting rooms, and the foyer. It is perhaps one of the distinctive characteristics of the clinic that so much can be accomplished in so small a space, while at the same time there is no feeling of overcrowding or unpleasantness. These features are conducive to good morale and satisfaction in the work that is being done.

FINANCE AND GENERAL ORGANIZATION

The unit was built in 1959 from funds provided by the Regional Hospital Board at a cost of about £150,000 ($420,000) including furnishings and equipment.

In 1964 the extension was completed to give more space for day patients. When it was planned an opportunity was afforded to invite cooperation from the university and from the Mental Health Association. This combined financing led to the setting up of a new records department for the Aberdeen Mental Hospital Group and to the establishment of the Ashgrove Club for rehabilitation.

It is an interesting reflection on the present organization of the National Health Service that collaboration with other institutions such as the university and with voluntary bodies, is both feasible and actively encouraged. Experience at the Ross Clinic has shown that there is no major obstacle to collaboration between state and voluntary organizations, particularly in the promotion of new or experimental services.

The organization of the clinic is therefore primarily the responsibility of the Regional Hospital Board insofar as overall policies are concerned. The Board of Management for the Aberdeen Mental Hospitals is responsible for its day-to-day administration and management. The professor of mental health of the university, who holds an honorary post with the hospital board, is the clinical director of the unit and his staff hold key appointments in it. Other consultant psychiatrists, holding appointments with the Regional Hospital Board, are attached to the clinic and are autonomous in relation to their clinical work, their patients, and their supporting staff.

STAFFING

Medical Staff

Medical staff are recruited from several sources as follows:

The University:
1. The professor of mental health—honorary clinical director.
2. Senior lecturer—honorary consultant psychiatrist.
3. Lecturer—honorary senior registrar.
4. Assistant lecturer—clinical psychologist.

Regional Hospital Board:
1. The deputy director—full-time consultant with the Regional Hospital Board who also has duties in the domiciliary service and links with the local health authority, and is the physician superintendent of Woodlands Home for Mentally Defective Children.
2. One part-time consultant psychiatrist who works four sessions with outpatients at the Ross Clinic, has other sessions in the Royal Mental Hospital and some sessions in private practice.
3. One consultant psychiatrist who divides his time between the Royal Mental Hospital and the Ross Clinic, where he is responsible for both inpatients and outpatients, and private practice.

4. Two senior registrars who are actively engaged in inpatient, day patient, and outpatient work. One of these has made a special study of the therapeutic community and is in charge of these activities in the new extension.

5. Two registrars in training.

6. Two house officers.

Medical Auxiliaries

1. One senior psychiatric social worker who also holds an honorary appointment with the university.

2. One psychiatric social worker post vacant at present.

3. One principal clinical psychologist.

4. One psychologist.

5. One probationer psychologist.

6. Two occupational therapists.

7. One art therapist.

In addition to the staff listed above, there are attendances from most other medical, psychological, and social worker staff on a session basis. In all there are 31 psychiatrists who attend the Ross Clinic at least once a week. These include all the senior and junior staff of Kingseat; most of those at the Royal Mental Hospital; and the consultants at Ladysbridge, Bilbohall, and the child psychiatry department. Thus there is a routine and built-in system of interaction and communication among all psychiatrists and ancillary staff in the region and the clinic acts as the hub of the service and the clearinghouse for professional exchanges (see Figure 4).

Nursing Staff

The nursing staff is provided largely from the main hospital and comes under the overall administration of the matron of the Royal Mental Hospital. An assistant matron and three nursing sisters are at the Ross Clinic, together with four staff nurses, eight student nurses, and two assistant nurses. Student nurses attend for a period of six to eight weeks, being in training at the Royal Mental

Hospital, at Kingseat, and also at the Royal Infirmary. The visiting staff includes physicians, surgeons, and others from the Royal Infirmary. Anesthetists attend routinely for E.C.T. from the main base in the Royal Infirmary.

THE TEAM SYSTEM

In accordance with the recommendations of the Platt Report and in keeping with many developments in both psychiatry and general medicine throughout the country, the medical, nursing, and ancillary staffs are now organized on the team principle.

For inpatients there are two teams, each responsible for one-half of the patients. There are two consultants, a senior registrar, a registrar, and a house official in each team, which has twice-weekly conferences attended by senior and junior nurses, occupational and art therapists, psychiatric social workers, and clinical psychologists. Each team is entirely responsible for the clinical policy relating to the patients assigned to it. Admission procedure is controlled by a senior consultant, either by direct referral if urgent, or through a waiting list. Assignment of new patients to a particular team is usually at random. If there has been previous contact with a particular team member, continuity of care is maintained.

With the aim of intensifying therapeutic activities in group settings and to provide for a large number of day patients, a third team has recently been established. Nominally under the direction of a consultant, the third team consists of a senior registrar, three selected trained nurses, and the occupational and art therapists. This team is responsible for the organization and operation of almost all the group activities of the clinic, except for actual group therapy conducted independently by other staff members. These activities include conventional but varied occupational therapy; art therapy; "self-help" groups contributing to the actual operation of the clinic (preparation and serving of meals, helping infirm patients, shopping, etc.); recreations; social activities of all kinds; and therapeutic meetings.

Where group treatment seems most appropriate, patients are

transferred to the group team. Both day patients and inpatients are assigned to this team from the other two in conference. For each patient a "prescription" is worked out by the team actually in charge of the case and in consultation with the group team members. The experiment has not operated long enough to make evaluations but it is considered at this stage that a more efficient utilization of staff skills and interests is achieved by this method.

It should be pointed out that the scheme was devised after it was realized that the physical layout of the clinic, even with the new extension, did not lend itself to a clear split between day patient and inpatient care. There is much common ground between these two groups of patients with regard to both treatment procedures and day-to-day administration. Accordingly, they were grouped together and a distinction of a different kind was established which dealt mainly with the extent to which interpersonal and social therapies are needed. Those requiring primarily individual investigation and treatment are assigned mainly to the first two teams and those requiring primarily group approaches are assigned to the new team.

The outpatient service is organized along rather similar lines but not so rigorously. There is a consultant with usually two assistants in attendance at each outpatient session when three, or perhaps four, new patients are examined. Each team arranges the examination and reporting on new patient referrals in its own way but reports are addressed to the referring source over the signature of the consultant in charge of the outpatient team.

Ultimate responsibility for the investigation and treatment of patients lies with the consultants who delegate duties to the senior registrars, registrars, and house officers. Generally speaking, the senior registrars act as second in command to the consultants and may carry out consultant duties in the latter's absence. Registrars undertake routine investigations and a fair proportion of the more straightforward physical and psychological treatments. House officers are mainly responsible for physical examination, routine case-taking, and special physical investigations.

ADMISSION PROCEDURES

Possibly the most distinctive feature of the admission procedure to the clinic (and more recently to other units in the region) is the initial interviewing of all patients referred to all the facilities. The case record now in general use contains a printed cover sheet in which can be entered extensive personal, social, and identifying data for use by the clinician, the hospital administration for operational studies, and the research unit for more fundamental epidemiological and sociological studies. At first contact and before the first psychiatric interview, the patient and/or his relative are interviewed for 20–30 minutes by specially trained staff who complete the forms. The basic training of these interviewers is clerical. They are selected for their warmth and maturity of personality and capacity to acquire the special training in reliable documentation that forms the essential core of their skill. It has been found that those with no psychiatric knowledge or sophistication are the most suitable, since they can approach their task without clinical involvement, neither prying into the personal and clinical aspects of the case nor giving any indication that this is what they might do. So far there has been only one refusal in over two thousand interviews—a figure that would not have been improved upon had the interviewers possessed psychiatric training.

The types of cases admitted for inpatient treatment are indicated in Table V. It will be noted that affective disorders and neurotic reactions form the majority and that those suffering from organic or senile reactions are less commonly admitted. On the other hand, there is a proportion of schizophrenics who have been investigated and treated with reasonable success in this type of unit, indicating that severity of illness as such does not prevent admission. It is by no means the case that psychotically disturbed patients cannot be treated along with those less disturbed. Indeed, a certain mixing of types of cases maintains a high state of alertness and interest on the part of the staff and gives a more realistic direction of interest among the patients. Segregation of quiet neurotic and depressive patients in a small unit can lead to a rather precious gentility more

TABLE V. *All admissions to Ross Clinic inpatient unit, 1962*

	(a) By age and sex		
Age	Male	Female	Total
0–14	3	1	4
15–24	18	30	48
25–34	19	34	53
35–44	22	29	51
45–54	24	21	45
55–64	20	20	40
65–74	2	4	6
75 and over	1	5	6
Totals	109	144	253

	(b) By diagnosis and sex		
Diagnosis	Male	Female	Total
Schizophrenia	9	9	18
Manic depressive reaction	22	21	43
Involutional melancholia	0	3	3
Senile and presenile psychoses	2	4	6
Other psychoses	6	4	10
Alcoholism	5	2	7
Other drug addiction	2	1	3
Organic syndromes	6	2	8
Neuroses except depression	24	32	56
Neurotic depression	19	48	67
Personality and behavior disorders	10	11	21
Miscellaneous	4	7	11
Totals	109	144	253

reminiscent of a hotel and a tacit understanding between patients and staff is reached that "bad behavior" is out of place. Psychiatrically, this is the peace of death and is antitherapeutic.

It should be mentioned that many patients admitted to the

clinic are in all respects similar to those admitted to the Royal and Kingseat Hospitals. This is because the psychiatrists attached to the Ross Clinic tend to admit patients they have previously seen as outpatients and elsewhere, and psychiatrists from the other two units follow out the same policy of maintaining continuity of treatment. It is more simple and acceptable to the patient for a psychiatrist, who is seeing a patient for the first time and who is satisfied that hospital admission is necessary, to say, "I think you should come into my ward (or hospital). I will be able to look after you (or see you regularly) there."

INVESTIGATION AND TREATMENT

During the first 48 hours after admission, patients are usually confined to bed, allowing detailed physical investigations and examinations to be carried out in the simplest way. This also gives the patient the best chance to become accustomed to the unfamiliar surroundings of the hospital and protects him from too many random and often disturbing stimuli. For many of the more severely ill patients, it is also best to start treatment in a fairly regressed state. Finally, bed rest does provide an opportunity for observation by nursing staff which is not possible if the patient is up and about. This applies not only to the more serious symptoms, such as hallucinosis, but also to more subtle symptoms such as the physical manifestations of anxiety.

Patients are not given sedative drugs, at least on the first night. This again gives the staff an opportunity to discover something about the patient's sleep pattern. This may be continued for a longer period, or perhaps even indefinitely. Every effort is made to prevent patients being sedated routinely. However, this is not a successful policy mainly because almost every patient coming into the hospital or outpatient clinic is already on sedatives, tranquilizers, or antidepressants.

Physical examination and investigations are of a fairly routine kind. Additional investigations, such as electroencephalography, and metabolic and body fluid studies, may be ordered. The laboratory services for the region are located in the respective university departments in the medical school only a few hundred yards away and all the specialist clinical services are available in the Royal Infirmary at about the same distance. Appropriate specialists are called in for other medical conditions, and occasionally patients are transferred to the general hospital for this purpose.

Psychiatric investigations follow a fairly conventional British pattern. The full case history is usually taken by the registrar and discussed at length by the consultant. All new patients are also discussed at the weekly team conferences and selected patients may be demonstrated in the lecture theater behind a one-way screen and tape recordings made. The psychodynamics may be formulated but the general climate of thought and practice in the clinic is eclectic.

Considerable emphasis is placed on social factors in relation to illness and here the psychiatric social worker and her colleagues, who are health visitors specially trained in mental health, make a valuable contribution in both investigation and treatment. Usually a case is not complete without a full report by one of the social worker staff.

Initial routine psychological investigations are of a fairly simple kind and include an intelligence test and the *Minnesota Multiphasic Personality Inventory*. Selected patients are referred to clinical psychology for more detailed investigation.

The EEG department has remained in the Royal Infirmary, still under the direction of the department of mental health, and providing a service for the whole hospital group. It is a little more inconvenient for patients to be sent up to the infirmary but the demand has not overwhelmed it. It is likely that the next step would be the setting up of a separate EEG department in the Royal Mental Hospital, serving all the psychiatric units in the region.

CONCLUSION

The original aims of the general hospital professorial unit were to promote the concept of early diagnosis and treatment of the more common psychiatric disorders, to establish functional contact with the general and mental hospital service on the one hand and the community welfare services on the other, and to establish optimal conditions for undergraduate and postgraduate teaching and research in the field of mental health. These have been at least partially realized. The academic department has been established at the center of the integrated service, has contributed significantly to its development, and has been as much concerned with the setting of high clinical standards as of initiating teaching programs and research, both operational and basic. It is considered that, for psychiatry, this central positioning of the department has advantages over the alternative plan of attachment of the academic unit as an appendage to the service, insulated from the day-to-day problems that face mental health workers and relatively remote from the point of action where breakdown occurs and where help must be given. It is also considered that much research sponsored by a peripheral or detached unit is vitiated by the absence of a genuine functional relationship between the patient and the research worker. There is no *quid pro quo* in the sense that the patient and his therapist do not seem to be benefiting in any tangible way from the procedures of investigation—possibly the reverse. Furthermore, in many types of inquiry in which case-finding is part of the procedure, the bringing to light of patients in need must be the first step in a therapeutic program and not mere fact-finding for its own sake, leaving the patient in the lurch at the very time he feels he requires assistance.

Role of the Mental Hospital

KINGSEAT: A LOCAL MENTAL HOSPITAL

Kingseat is one of two district mental hospitals which provide the bulk of adult psychiatric beds in the region (Figure 4). It was built in 1904 by the corporation of the city of Aberdeen to receive patients from the city. It was probably the first in Britain to be organized on the villa principle after a committee investigation of new mental hospital buildings, both at home and abroad. As there has been little building of mental hospitals since the turn of the century, it is one of the most modern in Scotland. The fact that it was evacuated during World War II to become a naval hospital accounts in part for the relative lack of overcrowding which is one of its distinctive features. In 1948 the administration of the hospital passed from the local authority to the Regional Board under the National Health Service (Scotland) Act of 1947.

There is accommodation for 810 patients in the wards and villas. Two single-story buildings house the admission unit and the geriatric unit. The 12 villas are two-story buildings with dormitories above and day rooms and a dining room below. In April 1962 a halfway house of 11 beds was opened in the city of Aberdeen.

Organization and Facilities

The chief officer of the hospital is the physician superintendent who is not only an administrator, but also has clinical charge of beds. Working with him in charge of the day-to-day running of the

617

hospital is the lay hospital secretary. Both of these are responsible to the Board of Management.

Medical staff consists of two consultants with seven junior doctors in various training grades, and one part-time assistant. Students are attached as paid clinical clerks. The medical staff is broadly organized in two teams under the two consultants, each of whom has responsibility for one of the male-female divisions of the hospital. The junior staff rotates between the two divisions. Consultant services in general medicine, surgery, gynecology, geriatrics, etc., are organized through the general hospitals in the city. A dental surgeon and an ophthalmologist visit regularly.

There are about one hundred male and one hundred female nurses, including student nurses, fully qualified registered mental nurses, enrolled nurses (nursing aides for whom there is now a register and some organized training), and nursing assistants who are untrained aides. A nurse training unit within the hospital, staffed by a qualified principal nursing tutor and an unqualified assistant tutor, conducts training. In addition to the nursing staff, there are the heads of the occupational therapy, work therapy, and social or recreational therapy departments, all of whom have experience in mental nursing. Ancillary staff includes a part-time psychologist and three social workers, headed by a trained psychiatric social worker.

The facilities for treatment of patients include a recently upgraded admission unit with mixed dining, lounge, and recreational areas, an electroconvulsive therapy suite, a small surgery room, and an art therapy room. The occupational therapy department can take about sixty patients at any one time and is mostly used for the craft work traditional to occupational therapy. Industrial contracts in the work therapy department are limited to the dismantling of general post office telephones and the stringing of paper carrier bags. The work therapist is also responsible for organizing patient occupation in the service departments of the hospital (grounds, kitchen, laundry, sewing room, etc.) and for work outside the hospital, mostly on farms. The social therapist has at his disposal a club room and a large recreation hall for the organization of social clubs, physical training classes, concerts, and cinema. He also runs various outdoor activities, such as bowling, tennis, and clock golf, bus tours, visits to theaters, and combined social club activities with the Royal Mental Hospital. "Radio Relay" puts out a hospital program to the villas twice weekly and attempts to keep patients informed and interested in the affairs of the hospital and encourages participation in them.

Intake

There is no official catchment area but largely because of historical association most patients come from the city of Aberdeen. The hospital also takes patients from the Shetland Islands, where it runs a quarterly clinic. A certain number are admitted from Aberdeen County and from Banffshire. The main route of referral of new patients is from general practitioners, via the regional mental health center, to the hospital. This ensures efficient screening and allows for the development of outpatient, domiciliary, and day hospital treatment. Unfortunately, the small hospital staff cannot find time to play as full a part in the regional psychiatric center as they might, and this does constitute something of a block between the general practitioner and the hospital. Referrals otherwise come from general practitioners directly; from the courts and probation officers; and, particularly in cases of re-referrals, from the hospital's own medical staff who are responsible for follow-up of discharged patients at the regional outpatient clinic.

Admissions cover the complete range of psychiatric illness— psychosomatic disorders, neuroses, depressive and schizophrenic reactions, senile states, and psychopathy. There is a loading, as one might expect, toward the more socially disabling illnesses. The total number of admissions remained very constant over the five to seven years up to 1962 when there were 542. In 1963, coincident with the introduction of informal admission under the Mental Health Act, there was a marked rise to 629 (Figure 4). The proportion of readmissions has risen steadily and in 1963 it was 55 per cent. This trend is common to most mental hospitals and the figure is only slightly above the national average. Despite the increased readmission rate the hospital population remains stable. Fifty per cent are discharged in six weeks or less, 70 per cent in three months or less, and 90 per cent in six months or less. This turnover takes place in roughly 15 per cent of the resident patients, the other 85 per cent being cases of long-term hospitalization. The geriatric problem is great, especially in the female division. Approximately 25 per cent of all admissions in 1963 were over the age of 65.

There has been some change in diagnostic composition with an increase in the percentage of what might broadly be called behavior disorders, such as psychopaths and alcoholics. A rough indication is given by figures for male admissions in the first four months of 1963:

Behavior disorders	42%
Functional psychoses (schizophrenia, depression, manic depressive states)	42%
Organic reactions	10%
Neuroses	5%

The full effect of the Mental Health Act, which came into operation on June 1, 1962, has yet to be felt. Indeed, fewer compulsorily detained patients have been admitted but this is accounted for mainly by the fact that patients without volition, such as in senile confusion states, can now be admitted informally at the request of their relatives.

Treatment

In general, all forms of therapy are accepted and applied as skills and resources allow, and treatment is not limited to the tenets of any one school. If there is any bias it is to what might broadly be called "social" therapy. Emphasis is on the development of human relations, by both medical staff and nurses. The value of relationship formation with lay members of hospital staff, such as tradesmen, is not excluded, but as yet little has been done with the formal manipulation of these in the therapeutic milieu.

THE ADMISSION UNIT. The most noticeable changes in atmosphere and attitude have taken place in the admission units of mental hospitals. Initially these were largely due to the therapeutic optimism aroused by the introduction of new forms of treatment, such as deep insulin coma therapy and E.C.T.; and, more recently, the psychotropic drugs. The more widespread use of voluntary admission in the 1930's induced a much less repressive attitude. The custodial tradition implied that the patient should be stripped physically of his clothing and mentally of his personality to suppress any tendency to disturbed behavior. This practice was not acceptable to the voluntary patient, and changes in attitudes came rapidly when there was some evidence that procedures were available which could bring benefit to the patient.

A second stage in the encouragement of patients to accept early treatment was initiated at Kingseat after the 1939-1945 war by the setting up of a "neuroses unit" to which only mildly disturbed patients were admitted. This was an open ward with active treatment where an attempt was made to preserve the patient's personality. Some of the good was negated by the fact that the adjoining ward was locked and contained compulsorily detained and highly disturbed patients. It was an ever-present threat of incarceration to the patients in the neuroses unit.

Since the introduction of the tranquilizers, it has been possible to control rapidly most psychotic behavior, and over the last two years all patients have been admitted to the same ward. There has been little evidence that this has caused any major upset to those less disturbed.

In the admission unit the main therapeutic endeavor is with physical treatments such as electroconvulsive therapy and the psychotropic drugs. There is also considerable psychotherapeutic support, explanation, and uncovering, though the amount of psychotherapy is limited by staff shortage. In addition, emphasis is placed upon the role of the nursing staff, both in support and in relationship formation. Nurses are taken very fully into the confidence of the medical staff. They are allowed access to patients' notes which are kept in the wards, and their opinions sought on patients' progress. The senior nursing staff in particular are encouraged to make and maintain good human relationships with their patients. More formal patient assignment nursing and more formal group discussions with the nursing staff are hampered by lack of staff and constant instability of the staff structure.

Ancillary aids to the understanding and treatment of the patient include psychological assessment and encouragement of self-expression in the art therapy department. Stimulation of constructive activity is of great importance and patients are encouraged to use the occupational therapy and work therapy departments. Here again the emphasis is as much on relationship formation as on the stimulation of activity.

Efforts are directed toward the preservation of the patient's personality. In particular, patients are expected to maintain a normal level of responsibility and conduct with the minimum use of repressive measures. A further aid is participation in the social life of the hospital and maintenance of outside contacts. Only in very exceptional cases are relatives asked to abstain from visiting and usually they are encouraged to visit as frequently as possible from the time of admission. Patients are allowed home on weekend leave as soon as possible.

THE LONG-STAY WARDS. The opportunity for active treatment of the recently admitted patient and the relative failure of the long-stay patient to respond to physical treatments formerly led to a concentration of medical interest in the admission unit. This trend has now been partly reversed by the ethical consideration that it is wrong that patients should be abandoned, and also by the practical consideration that one cannot have a therapeutic atmosphere in one part of the hospital while the rest of it is neglected, for it is the total atmosphere which determines the therapeutic efficiency of each part. Use of psychotropic drugs extended rapidly throughout the hospital, prompted to a certain extent by the demands of nursing staff for exhibition of these drugs which undoubtedly control disturbed behavior. However, it could be seen readily that, though the gross manifestations of psychotic behavior were lessened, the patient could not be cured unless further measures were taken. The picture in the chronic wards had changed from one of restless, disturbed impulsiveness to one of widespread anergy.

It was realized that only the nursing staff could help here and they were encouraged to stimulate the patient's activity. Greater use was made of the hospital's maintenance and garden departments for the employment of patients, and occupational and work therapy were encouraged on the wards. Generally, there is now greater patient activity and alertness and a notable increase in sociability. The work and social therapies were also used to develop human relationships between staff and patients. In some of the villas patients were divided into smaller groups and made the special responsibility of individual nurses. Here again, this could have gone further and become more effective if adequate nursing staff had been available. The most important achievement to date is that there has been a steady evolutionary change in the attitudes of the nursing staff. To some extent they have been able to overcome their traditional custodial attitudes and adopt a more friendly and less repressive approach.

It is difficult to assess just how successful these measures have been in relation to discharge of long-term patients from hospital. Though there is no doubt at all that the total atmosphere has become therapeutically active and optimistic, we have no evidence that the mental hospital population will realize the expectation of the English Ministry of Health plan for the future development of mental health services based on a major reduction in the number of hospital beds required.

Discharge and Follow-up

It is considered that treatment in this hospital is for most patients only a phase in the total therapeutic program and that it may have been preceded by, and is likely to be followed by, outpatient and domiciliary care. Different forms of help can be offered at different points in illness, according to patients' psychological and social needs. In one sense, therefore, there is no "after-care," only "care" of various kinds, which is provided within the broad context of the community mental health services of which the hospital is an integral part.

All admissions are potential discharges but discharge is not an aim in itself. The aim is to make the patient sufficiently self-reliant to leave the hospital successfully and to modify the stresses to which he will be subject once he is out of hospital by providing support for him and his family through various agencies, principally those operated through the hospital social work department.

The assumption that every patient admitted is a potential discharge cannot be maintained in every case, particularly where mental symptoms are the result of degenerative or other organic cerebral disease. But even here care must be taken to ensure that the patient's relatives do not automatically assume that he will be hospitalized for the remainder of his life.

Visits by the social worker may precede the patient's first visit home, and she may also visit while he is home on a trial period prior to discharge. The attitudes of relatives and the adaptation of the patient are discussed between the social worker and the medical staff and decisions reached as to the next appropriate step in rehabilitation. It is of special importance to recognize that the process of readaptation may be long-term and that to hurry discharge before the patient is ready or before the relatives are ready fully to accept him will tend to lead to premature readmission.

Admission is very rarely refused, and *readmission* is seldom refused, because patients with long-term illness may have periods when, though by no means cured, they are sufficiently well to be out of hospital for a time, even though they can be expected to return sooner or later. The need for readmission often depends as much upon the diminishing tolerance of relatives as upon the recrudescence of the patient's symptoms. Through home visits by social workers and regular outpatient follow-up by medical staff at the regional outpatient center, an attempt is made to ensure that the patient is readmitted before relationships between him and his family deteriorate to the point at which mutual rejection seriously jeopardizes the possibilities of future rehabilitation.

A few patients are helped and encouraged to find and start regular work while continuing to live in the hospital, travelling back and forth each day. Unfortunately, this is restricted since the hospital is about twelve miles from Aberdeen and facilities for travelling in and out are not ideal. Another inhibiting factor, particularly for unskilled workers, is the high level of unemployment in the area.

A few informal patients leave against medical advice, but the great majority are discharged by arrangement with their hospital doctor after discussion with one of the consultants. In every case, a brief intimation of discharge is sent on the same or following day to the patient's family doctor, giving the salient features of the case, treatment while in hospital, and recommended treatment after discharge. At this time, too, arrangements are made for outpatient follow-up by the doctor principally concerned with his case in hospital and by a social worker at home.

SOCIAL WORK AND THE LOCAL HEALTH AUTHORITY. The supply of highly trained psychiatric social workers has never been sufficient to meet the demand, and in 1958 the hospital, although increasingly aware of the need for a follow-up service, was without anyone trained in this field. Various possibilities existed, such as the use of mental nurses for the purpose, but for several reasons, including a dawning awareness of the coming importance of local authority community care services, an approach was made to the Medical Officer of Health for the city of Aberdeen. A number of meetings were held with the physician superintendent of the hospital and an arrangement made whereby a specially chosen member of the local authority health visitor staff was assigned to deal with social problems, community care, and follow-up work. The worker was based on the hospital and entirely under the clinical direction of the physician superintendent and his staff, although continuing to be paid by the local authority.

The person originally chosen for this work had no previous experience of mental patients and the psychiatric social worker post was not filled until 1959. The health visitor then worked under her nominal supervision. A second full-time health visitor from the local authority was seconded in the same way in 1963 so that the hospital now has three full-time workers in the social work department, only one of whom, the psychiatric social worker, is an employee of the Regional Hospital Board.

Another venture with similar objects began in 1961 when two health visitors were assigned to the hospital for instruction and experience under the psychiatric social worker for two days a week over a period of six months. These were replaced by two others for the succeeding six months and the system has continued without a break. Thus, of the ordinary district health visitors, 12 have had experience and instruction designed to help them cope with psychiatric illness in their district. In 1963 a group of 24 student health visitors were given a week's intensive course of instruction at the hospital in all aspects of the care and treatment of the mentally ill.

In a few cases it has been found possible to pass on the domiciliary care of a patient to local authority mental welfare officers. This is likely to grow as these workers increase in numbers and gain in experience but follow-up and community care is handled at present almost exclusively by hospital staff except in relation to the Shetland Isles.

In the Shetlands, a mental health officer, working under the local medical officer of health, deals with all the domiciliary care and follow-up of patients discharged from Kingseat. While he is responsible officially only to the medical officer of health, he is frequently in direct communication with the hospital, attends all psychiatric outpatient clinics in Shetland, and spends about a week in the hospital two or three times a year to see Shetland patients, discuss his problems, and keep in touch with current methods.

Conclusion

Like the majority of mental hospitals in Britain, Kingseat is in the process of evolution. In some hospitals there have been apparently revolutionary changes in the treatment of the long-stay patient. The open-door policy, work in industrial therapy, and the use of groups have been introduced as a *tour de force*. At Kingseat it seems that the most important thing is to produce changes in attitude in the nursing staff rather than introduce revolutionary techniques. This is inevitably a slow process.

One of the greatest problems is the shortage of both medical and nursing staff. There are only two consultants, one of whom has considerable administrative responsibilities. The junior staff, being mostly in training grades, is absorbed in the pursuit of academic qualifications requiring time off for attendance at other clinics, lectures, and reading. They have little time to spare for involvement with "administrative therapies."

Many of the nursing staff live 12 miles away in the city of Aberdeen and have to work a 12-hour day. The working week has been reduced recently to 44 hours so that a group cannot be in contact with the same nurse throughout the week. Staff shortages are also increased by the long periods student nurses must spend away from the ward in "block" study at the nurses' training school. This is wholly desirable but combined with longer holidays, shorter hours, and sickness, it is very difficult to keep a stable staff on any one ward and the constant changes lessen nurse-patient contact.

The other major problem is the lack of facilities for rehabilitation. Units do not yet exist either within or outside the hospital where a patient can be stimulated and encouraged to perform a full day's work of the type that he will encounter upon discharge. At the moment no more than four to five hours of very simple work can be offered daily. When the patient comes to take up a job, he is not ready to work a full eight hours under normal industrial pressures. There is no rehabilitation center or sheltered workshop outside the hospital and as there is unemployment in the region, it is not easy to get employers to accept people whose work record is likely to be poor. However, there is hope for developments as local health authorities set up rehabilitation procedures under the new Mental Health Act.

Extension of all these services can be expected in the future, together with an improvement in the ability to use nursing staff in a psychotherapeutic role and an increasing sophistication in the training of junior medical staff, particularly in psychotherapeutic techniques.

BILBOHALL: THE PERIPHERAL UNIT

Even in a relatively small, compact, and well-organized area like the northeast of Scotland, with its centripetal lines of communication converging on the city of Aberdeen, it would be misleading to give the impression that societal homogeneity prevailed, or that integration of regional services automatically ensured parity of access. The inevitable concentration of services in the regional mental health center and its associated mental hospitals in and near the city emphasizes the social and geographical distance of the rural periphery. Community mental health implies services based within the social and geographical contexts of their catchment areas. It will be apparent that this represents a major reversal of the earlier policies of extrusion so graphically illustrated by the U.S. Joint Commission for Mental Illness and Health in the book *Action for Mental Health*.

The northeast was particularly fortunate in having already available a small mental hospital situated in the northerly part of the mainland. The following account of its history and present-day development illustrates several points of relevance to modern concepts of community mental health. For instance, the central theme of community responsibility for its own mentally ill in terms of rehabilitation is seen to date from the latter part of the nineteenth century. The "open door" and the concept of social and vocational therapy had been practiced even before the "extrusion" phenomenon took over. It may be that the cyclical fashions of psychiatry exemplified in the history of this small hospital reflect changes in community attitudes, tolerance levels and reactions, which are associated with wider changes in the social context, such as economic growth and stagnation, war and peace, and their concomitant value systems.

History

In 1819 a bequest of £20,000 from the late Dr. Alexander Gray of the East India Company, formerly a native of Elgin, founded Dr. Gray's Hospital, a general hospital for the sick poor of Elgin and district (Figure 1). Sixteen years later, the trustees of this hospital gave funds to the county authorities for the building of the Elgin and District Pauper and Lunatic Asylum. This was a small building adjacent to the general hospital and accommodated 12 lunatics in cells.

Statutory records were not kept until 1858 when the commissioners of the newly formed Board of Lunacy for Scotland began to inspect and report on all asylums throughout Scotland. In 1859, following their first visit to Elgin, they described it as "the most dismal asylum in Scotland." A number of critical, indeed disparaging, annual reports followed until in 1865, again with financial help from the trustees of Dr. Gray's Hospital, a new asylum building was completed. It is substantially the same building which is in use as the district mental hospital today.

Nineteenth-century treatment for mental illness was minimal. In one report it was noted that "no patients get medication for their mental disease." From 1835 until 1949 there was never a full time medical officer in charge of the hospital. Initially the asylum was administered by the keeper, and in the early twentieth century a lady superintendent was in charge. General practitioners serving in the district had part-time appointments as medical officers. In the early days there were numerous changes and lengthy spells when no medical officer was appointed. One reason was perhaps hinted at in a commissioners' report "that the District Board give serious consideration to increasing the remuneration of the medical officer."

THE ERA OF FREEDOM. In spite of minimal medical treatment, the hospital was a pioneer in anticipating the development of occupational and work therapy. In 1863 it was recorded that "23 lunatics of powerful build were zealously engaged in trenching or dragging lustily the roots of trees." Daily parole was in common use to permit patients to take up occupation or trade in Elgin itself.

In 1877 new locks were fitted throughout the hospital, making unnecessary the constant locking and unlocking of all doors, and the next year Bilbohall Farm of 130 acres was acquired for the occupation of the inmates. With 30 additional acres of asylum land this provided "a means of curative treatment productive of real benefit to both the bodily and mental health of the patients."

The open-door policy was increasingly adopted at the farm about a mile from the hospital, where "it has not been found necessary to adopt any special discipline." "None of the appliances usual in asylums for ensuring the detention of patients are to be seen; the patients are living in circumstances which have scarcely any resemblance to those of ordinary asylum life." Patients were also encouraged to work for neighboring farms, so that "the public are led to look without ignorant fears upon the inmates and the feeling is produced in the patients that they are still recognized as useful members of the community. The feeling that patients in asylums ought to be cut off from all dealings with the outer world is good neither for the patients nor for the outer world."

Opportunities for escape were abundant in this era of freedom from restriction, but only two absences without leave occurred in nine years. A principle of judicious seclusion was recognized and patients were found to be "in a state of tranquillity creditable to those in charge."

THE CUSTODIAL TRADITION.   In 1880 the hospital was enlarged, a high wall was built, and gradually the custodial role of an asylum with severance of links with the community took over from the former regime of freedom and liberty.

During the first half of the twentieth century the custodial tradition continued. Admissions were regulated by discharges and deaths, and the asylum was constantly overcrowded (Table VI). Gradually, however, links with the community were formed and patients began to attend the local movie theater in the era of the "talkies" and also local parish churches. The hospital enjoyed the advantage of close proximity to the town and district from which its patients were drawn. There were good lines of communication and close cooperation with the adjoining general hospital.

TABLE VI. *Bilbohall Hospital: Numbers of beds and patients, 1835–1963*

Year	No. of beds officially approved	No. of patients
1835	12	14
1865	75	92
1890	100	104
1910	150	169
1940	175	192
1960	200	216
1963	212	185–200

From Asylum to Hospital—The National Health Service

The National Health Service came into operation in 1948. The following year the physician superintendent of the neighboring county asylum at Banff was given a joint appointment with Elgin Asylum, the names of the institutions changing to Ladysbridge Hospital, Banff, and Bilbohall Hospital, Elgin. Thus, close contact with a physician trained in the treatment and care of the mentally ill was ensured. Physical methods of treatment were introduced and intensified and for the first time some use was made of voluntary admission. Although this had been possible in Scotland since the nineteenth century, very few voluntary entries had taken place in Elgin until 1949. The average annual number of admissions in the 1920's and 1930's was around 14 patients. In the 1950's it progressed through 20 to 50 admissions per annum.

The Regional Mental Health Service

In 1954 the first district outpatient service was offered in the adjacent general hospital. Attendances in the first three years

averaged 85. With the inception of the regional psychiatric service
in Aberdeen, monthly visits to Elgin by a senior and junior member
of the Ross Clinic staff initiated a service for follow-up and for new
patient referrals. By 1961 three members of the Ross Clinic were
attending on one different day each week to conduct outpatient
clinics at the general hospital and outpatient and inpatient care in
Bilbohall Hospital. Closer links were established with the regional
service by regular visits of a clinical psychologist, an art therapist,
and other ancillary staff.

This extension of the regional psychiatric services from the center
to the periphery was inevitable. With the advent of modern techniques and diminishing prejudice of the public and medical practitioners leading to an increased referral rate, it became more
necessary for the specialist to go out to the periphery rather than
have patients from the periphery come into the center.

At this time also the local Board of Management was engaged in
the administrative integration of Dr. Gray's and Bilbohall Hospitals.
Since 1948 nursing services, particularly in training, have been inter-
changeable. The nurse tutor serves both hospitals. The mental
hospital had long made use of medical and surgical services in the
general hospital. In 1959 a group matron for Dr. Gray's and Bilbohall was appointed. Finally a full-time physician superintendent
was appointed to Bilbohall Hospital in 1963.

The Peripheral Community Mental Health Center

Today Bilbohall Hospital has 100 male and 112 female beds.
Compulsorily detained patients number only 21 (10 male and 11
female) and bed occupancy is variable (Table VI). It is recognized
that to offer a full mental health service to the community, beds
must be readily available. Intensive efforts are made to discharge
patients when improved and to ensure that no misplacement occurs.
In 1881 the commissioners commented, "The number of patients in
a district asylum always depends to some extent on the amount of
energy shown by parochial officials in providing for such of the
harmless and incurable patients as are suitable for treatment at
home, in private dwellings or in parish accommodation." This

principle of the right patient in the right bed is enforced today, but is dependent on close cooperation with general practitioner services, general hospital services, and local authority medical and welfare services. Exchanges with the regional mental deficiency service of mentally subnormal patients without emotional illness for those with predominantly mental illness have reduced the number of mentally subnormal patients at present in Bilbohall to 21, only 8 of whom are rated as priority for transfer.

In the past the hospital was divided structurally into a male and female hospital, each with its respective combined sick and admission ward and numerous long-stay dormitories. Now, with building upgrading and reorganization, essential units are structurally identified and independently staffed according to their needs. On the male and female sides there are admission units with 20 beds each, geriatric units (35 beds), and long-stay units (50 beds).

Inpatient service is provided for a population of 90,000 and outpatient service for 60,000. Clinics are held at both Bilbohall and Dr. Gray's Hospitals. Banff, the neighboring county town, has its own outpatient clinic in the general hospital in Banff. Since 1962 day-patient facilities have been offered and with an intensive rehabilitation and resocialization program, an increasing number of "long kept" and potential long-stay patients can be discharged to the community. Readmission policy is liberal and the "revolving door" has replaced the "open door."

In the community, psychiatric outpatient follow-up is increasingly used, together with local authority home-visiting and close liaison with general practitioners. The latter is much more readily obtained and maintained in a rural than in an urban area. A close link with the community is maintained through the "League of Friends," a group of voluntary workers and representatives of voluntary organizations. This is an important means of community education and information-giving.

Conclusion

The reinstatement of older ideas in a new and technically more sophisticated age brings with it new methods for their achievement.

The pattern of services now existing in Elgin and district bears a remarkable resemblance to the comprehensive community mental health center proposed by President Kennedy in 1963. Indeed, the description of such centers given by Felix (1) could hardly be more apposite to Bilbohall:

Such a Center would be more broadly based than either the traditional out-patient clinic or the usual State institution, and would be the pivot of future mental health activities within the community. It would be close to the patient's home, and would provide preventive services, diagnostic services, out-patient and in-patient treatment, and transitional and rehabilitation services. As his needs change, the patient in such a Center would more quickly move to other appropriate services. Basically, he would be able to proceed from diagnosis to cure and rehabilitation. Other essential services provided by the Center would be consultative, educational and informational services to the public and professional persons. Skilled Community Mental Health staff would be available to help physicians, teachers, clergymen, police and probation officers, lawyers and social agency personnel deal with the mental health problems of those they face in their day-to-day work.

REFERENCE

1. Felix, R. H. *New Directions in Community Mental Health Services.* Paper prepared for Horizon House's 11th Annual Community Meeting, Philadelphia, 1963.

Services for Special Groups

GERIATRICS

In considering geriatric patients, it is necessary to touch on general as well as psychiatric services, because there is much overlap. Wilson *et al.* (7) have drawn attention to the frequency with which more than one pathology is found in elderly people. In 200 consecutive admissions, three-quarters of whom were over 70 years old, they found an average of six separate pathologies per patient. In the elderly it is common to find either a psychiatric condition secondary to physical disease or physical disease and mental disorder coexistent but not directly related. It is obvious that misplacement may easily occur, a patient more suited to a general geriatric ward being admitted to a psychiatric hospital and vice versa. Kidd (4), and others have recently drawn attention to the frequency of such misplacement but it is equally clear that to some extent any unit dealing with geriatric patients should be prepared for both physical and mental symptomatology and disease, and the planning of services for the elderly should be comprehensive.

Elderly people here are defined as those who have attained their sixty-fifth birthday. Biologically there is little justification for fixing any arbitrary demarcation; a person is as old as he looks and feels and this is often the best clinical guide, but for planners, statisticians, and administrators, such unnatural tricks are necessary. Age 65 is a major social landmark in our culture, for it is the age at which men retire and qualify for the old age pension. Anomalously the age for women is 60. This end of an epoch in a man's life demands a complete readjustment which may precipitate psychiatric ill health.

The Geriatric Population

In the 1951 Scottish census, 10.9 per cent of the population of the northeast region, or 52,300 people, were aged 65 and over. Females over 65 constituted a slightly larger proportion of all females at around 12 per cent. The ratio of females to males ranged from 1.64 for Aberdeen City, to 1.29 for Aberdeen County. Figures for the country as a whole are similar. However, in the Orkney and Shetland Islands, the proportions of females over 65 were 15.9 per cent and 17.7 per cent, respectively. The higher percentage of old people in Orkney and Shetland is almost certainly due to emigration of the younger age groups.

Provisions for the Care of the Elderly

Elderly people requiring psychiatric inpatient treatment or who grow old with psychiatric conditions in hospital are cared for in three mental hospitals. In 1955 there were 614 elderly patients in psychiatric beds in the region.

There were 877 designated general geriatric beds, nearly three-quarters of which are under the direction of a central geriatric unit with its headquarters in Aberdeen and beds in seven peripheral hospitals in Aberdeenshire, Moray, and Banff. About 16 per cent are for assessment and rehabilitation, the remaining 84 per cent for long-term care. There are also some 30 beds in Shetland which are regularly used for geriatric patients, about one-half of them for long-term convalescence. The general hospitals also carry a proportion of patients over 65, who are acutely ill.

For those whose social circumstances and personality resources conspire to make a continued life of self-sufficiency in the community impossible, the local health authorities and various voluntary organizations, such as the churches and the Old People's Welfare Council, provide a number of "Eventide" homes. There are 438 places available in Aberdeen City, 277 in the county, 111 in Banffshire, 49 in Kincardine, 106 in Moray, 42 in Shetland, and 80 in Orkney. This amounts to an overall availability of 1103 places or 21 per 1000 population over 65, of which three-quarters are under local authorities. Thus, of a geriatric population of 52,000, 600 are in mental hospitals, 900 are in general geriatric beds, and 1100 are in old folks' homes. This is a total of 5 per cent who are in some institution, compared with an estimated 6 per cent for Scotland as a whole. What proportion of the geriatric population living in the community would go to hospitals or old folks' homes if more facilities were available is not known. The situation is probably not homogeneous throughout the region. Any study of waiting lists is misleading, because if vacancies are very limited, doctors do not use them but, rather, wait until their patients become emergencies.

Community services are not uniform throughout the region, but in places are very good. In Orkney, for example, much progress has been made following a sample survey by Richardson, Brodie, and Wilson (8). The importance of social isolates as potential mental casualties has been recognized and there are now very few old people living alone. The general standard of housing has been much improved by special building for the elderly in the two principal towns. There is a comprehensive chiropody service and three geriatric health visitors are employed by the local authority to visit regularly everyone over age 65. In Aberdeen City any old person who comes to the attention of the local health authority is recorded in a register and health visitors continue to maintain contact unless expressly asked not to do so.

Psychogeriatric Patients at the Royal Mental Hospital

At the end of 1955 there were 1011 patients in the hospital, of whom 333 were age 65 or over. Only about 25 per cent of males but 40 per cent of females were in the geriatric age range.

Schizophrenia (*300*)* and paranoia (*303*) together accounted for

---

* Italic numbers in parentheses are codes from the *International Statistical Classification of Diseases*, Sixth Revision.

33 per cent of this group. A further 17 per cent were labelled depression (301) or involutional melancholia (302). Thus just about one-half the elderly residents were suffering from functional psychoses. Senile psychoses (304), presenile psychoses (305), and arteriosclerotic dementia (306) together accounted for 37 per cent of the elderly group.

One reflection prompted by these findings is that the image of geriatric psychiatric nursing as very onerous calling concerned mainly with demented people is false. As things stood here in 1955, this was not half the problem.

Only 10 per cent of geriatric patients had been in hospital for less than six months, over three-quarters had been in for two years or more and half had been in for ten years and more. This suggests that a unit admitting geriatric psychiatric cases for assessment or treatment and disposal would need to be backed by three times its number of chronic beds. This is in accordance with the experience of Robinson (9) at the Crichton Royal, Dumfries, who handles all geriatric admissions in two acute wards of 20 beds each, backed by two long-stay wards of 60 beds each.

None of the 95 patients with schizophrenia had been in hospital less than six months, 70 per cent had been in for over twenty years and almost 90 per cent for over ten years. Only 2 patients suffering from paranoia out of 14 had been hospitalized less than six months and 10 for over ten years.

Of 57 patients with depressive psychoses (301 and 302), only 4 had been retained for less than six months, 4 for less than two years; and the rest were long-stay, 39 of whom had been hospitalized for over ten years. Such a large number of depressives who have apparently failed to respond to treatment (E.C.T. is freely given at the Royal Mental Hospital), might at first sight surprise and disappoint, but it accords well within Post's findings in his follow-up study of affective illness in old age (7). Using criteria not only of mental symptoms, but also of social adjustment and duration of incapacity, he found that in only 19 per cent were there no detrimental long-term effects, a further 35 per cent were able to live tolerable lives in spite of subsequent, sometimes protracted periods of mental illness, and the remaining 46 per cent suffered a sustained decline, which was severe in 18 per cent. He also found that the type of treatment did not influence the long-term results.

Of the demented (*304, 305, 306*), one-half had been in for less than two years, and a little over 20 per cent for less than six months. Nonetheless, 17 patients out of 124 in this group were still alive after five years and 9 after ten years.

There are 14 female and 10 male wards in the hospital. A census at August 28, 1963, gave a picture of how elderly patients were distributed about the hospital. On the female side, 20 per cent was the lowest proportion in any ward; four wards had 20–29 per cent; six between 30 and 60 per cent; and four over 60 per cent of elderly patients, one of these having 90 per cent. The picture on the male side was rather different. The male admission ward and the male disturbed ward had only 3 per cent each of elderly patients. Four of the wards contained between 20 per cent and 29 per cent of old people, one 50 per cent, and one 80 per cent. Thus there was a tendency to concentrate the male geriatric patients in two wards. Whether segregation of elderly patients is to their advantage is debatable. There are arguments for and against but the special needs of individuals should not be submerged by too rigid administrative generalizations and planning. The physical and mental state of the individual will probably always be the best guide as to what sort of ward he should be in. Perhaps the wide dispersion of elderly patients is not unassociated with the fact that nearly 80 per cent have been hospitalized for over two years and 50 per cent are suffering from functional psychoses. They may well have grown old in a particular ward and there has been no physical or mental reason to move them on reaching the magic age of 65.

In 1962, about 20 per cent of 600 admissions to the Royal Mental Hospital were age 65 or over. With 11 per cent of the general population age 65 and over, this is consistent with the expectation that the chances of being admitted to a mental hospital are increased in the senium.

In those female wards containing largely geriatric patients, there are from four to five patients per nurse. The male ward with 80 per cent of geriatric cases has only one nurse for eight patients. As Exton-Smith *et al.* (1) point out, bedridden elderly women are very much more time-consuming and difficult to nurse than bedridden elderly men.

The most obvious staff deficiency is in social work. The Royal Mental Hospital has only one psychiatric social worker with no assistants. The County of Aberdeen local health authority has recently started social worker visits to discharged patients but there is no hospital contact with these social workers and they have no knowledge of the patient in hospital. There is no social worker with a special interest in geriatric psychiatry.

The Grounds for Change

There is often a body of people who like things as they are and cannot see why any change at all should be necessary. Changes inevitably cost money and there is no certainty that new methods will be any more successful than the old. There is a golden rule for the exponents of change which is often neglected. The experiment, for that is what it is, should be designed in such a way that hypotheses can be tested and clear answers can be obtained as to whether or not the innovations are useful.

There are *a priori* grounds for urging changes. The physical surroundings in which many geriatric patients are now confined are esthetically displeasing. The majority of old people would rather stay at home than go into any sort of institution, so when they have to go into one, they should find it as much like home as possible. Large, crowded, dingy wards and segregation of the sexes are unnatural. Such places must often frighten relatives and discourage their maintaining a close tie with their old folk, and this in turn increases the difficulty of getting elderly people home again. Where this difficulty is due to mistaken attitudes of relatives, not enough is done by staff to modify them. Some staff attitudes could also be altered with profit. Even today, for example, there is reluctance among some nursing staff to get elderly patients out of bed. It may seem to require more time and effort to get them up, and staff may be short. There may be the fear that they will fall and injure themselves; or the idea that they will be warmer and more comfortable in bed; or the lack of up-to-date equipment such as walking aids. There are wards in the Royal Mental Hospital where sheer lack of space and failure of heating in winter makes it impossible to get the aged out of bed.

Plans for Improvement

What sort of service should we plan for? Robinson (9) advocated a domiciliary visit to every patient prior to admission, either by the psychiatrist or by a hospital social worker. This not only afforded insight into the home conditions, but also gave an opportunity to explain to relatives that the patient was coming into the hospital only temporarily in the first instance and might well return home. For a variety of reasons, people may delay until their elderly relatives have become an insuperable burden at home and when at last they are forced to call for help they may want no more to do with this care.

An admission unit for geriatric psychiatric patients seems desirable where assessment can take place, treatment be instituted, and in many cases some route out of the hospital be followed. The first hope is always that the patient can go home. Here the general practitioner will command the situation, but he will require assistance from local authority services; visits from the district nurse may be necessary for physical disabilities and social worker visits are likely to benefit the psychiatric aspects. Ideally there would be consultation in hospital between the physician in charge and the various people who will be looking after the patient when he gets home, but in a widespread district this is usually impossible. In practice the best that can be obtained is a full explanatory letter.

Day hospital care may be helpful where inactivity at home threatens to lead to reactive depression. Woodford-Williams *et al.* (12) have described their experiences in a thoughtful and well-planned study with careful attention to controls. By having patients attend one day a week they were able to treat 168 patients with facilities each day for only 25 to 30. They found a significantly reduced rate of "depression" in the treated group. In this region, day hospital care would only be useful for those who live in or near the few larger towns.

A number of elderly patients, after a short stay in hospital, are neither really well enough to look after themselves at home nor, by reason of their eccentricities, very suitable for the usual type of old folks' home nor ill enough to remain in a mental hospital. For such patients there seems to be a gap which might be filled by some form of hostel with minimal supervision and emphasis on self-help and mutual cooperation.

After assessment some geriatric psychiatric patients will have to be transferred to a geriatric hospital because of physical illness. Finally, there will be a residue who will have to remain for the rest of their lives in a mental hospital. Of these, some will be more or less bedridden and will require heavy nursing, and some will be ambulant. Both groups should be in many small units rather than in a few large ones. For the ambulant there is much to commend the homely atmosphere of mixed wards with as much single accommodation as possible. It may be necessary at times to lock a few doors since wandering is such a common expression of senile organic changes and tactful restraint is essential.

Conclusion

The care of the old is seen as primarily a community problem. Those in need must be discovered and assessed in their homes before they are past help. After hospitalization the path back to their homes must be aided in every way possible. Thus the most important figure must always be the general practitioner though he can be tremendously assisted by various local authority services.

The key to success in the treatment of the elderly must surely be flexibility and general competence. A multiplicity of pathologies must be expected and nobody who is only an expert in a narrow field is suited to this work. A geriatric psychiatrist must feel at home with physical disease just as the general physician must be able to contain a degree of mental abnormality, so that the unfortunate old patient is spared a restless shuffling back and forth from one unit to another and from one physician to another. Nonetheless, every physician has his limitations and when he needs his colleagues' help, it must be easily and quickly available. The closest liaison must exist, therefore, between the geriatric psychiatrist and the geriatric physician. Such liaison is always most satisfactory at a personal level and, in this respect, a center the size of Aberdeen is especially blessed. It is large enough to support competent people in all the major specialties, yet small enough for all to have a nodding acquaintance with each other and to feel a regional loyalty.

MENTAL DEFICIENCY

The mental deficiency services for the region are based on two main centers. The largest is Ladysbridge Hospital, Banff, and the other, for children, is at Woodlands Home near Aberdeen (Figure 4). Ladysbridge caters to all mental defectives over the age of 16. At present it houses 338 patients but is being enlarged and building will be carried on continuously through 1969 until a total of 515 beds are available, including a children's unit of 25 beds for the use of patients living on the south side of the Moray Firth.

Community care and adequate social rehabilitation are the main objects of present policy. To achieve this it must first be ensured that the hospital itself is an accepted part of the community and is not separated from it physically nor by any emotional barriers which could result from fear or ignorance. Second, if patients are going to become either totally or partially self-supporting members of society, realistic work and behavior values must be adopted for training programs, such as exist in the world outside.

The Hospital in the Community

The first of these aims can be achieved if the hospital is conscious of the surrounding community and develops its own public relations scheme toward it. Maximum contact between patients and their relatives and friends in the community is encouraged by allowing daily visiting in both mornings and afternoons. Local groups, such as churches and guilds, are invited to see the hospital and its activities. Such visits led to the formation of the very active League of Friends, who fill an important gap by providing a regular visiting service for patients who have no relatives. Visitors are encouraged to take patients for outings in the adjoining towns, so that they do not feel that the hospital authorities are trying to isolate them.

Another means is through liaison with the local authority. Outpatient clinics for defectives are held in the local authority premises in Banff. The education authority's occupation center and special school at Banff are visited regularly by medical staff from the hospital. All student nurses, as part of their routine training, spend at least a month working in the occupation center and a month in the special school. This has made it possible to admit younger people to Ladysbridge and send them to the special school in Banff daily. Thus the child continues to receive education which would otherwise be impossible and education authority staff are more willing to take a difficult child for a trial period knowing that he is receiving adequate treatment and supervision. Indeed schoolteachers now give medication to patients at appropriate intervals while at school. The social worker is employed three days a week by the hospital and two days by Banff County Council. He provides first-class communication and helps both hospital and local authority services to be aware of the other's problems.

Outpatient clinics are held weekly at the Ross Clinic in Aberdeen and in Elgin. Approximately every quarter, the large orphanage at Aberlour in Banffshire, where a number of subnormal children are boarded out, is visited to discuss difficulties with the rector and to give guidance on points of day-to-day management. Children needing more specific therapy attend one of the clinics. The clinics themselves play a useful part in the scheme by acting as a sympathetic platform on which relatives can discuss their problems. They allow advice to be given to parents on training, especially on the order in which it should be attempted in any particular case. They provide a place where simple psychotherapy and counselling can be carried out with older subnormals and a useful method of keeping down the readmission rate by routine frequent follow-up of rehabilitated patients. Difficulties can be discussed and cleared up before they become insoluble problems for the patient.

Considerable numbers of domiciliary visits are undertaken with patients in their own and in local authority homes throughout the area. The majority of hospital admissions in subnormals are precipitated by social factors and it is difficult to decide on priorities fairly unless one has good insight into the conditions in the individual patient's home.

By maintaining community contact and stressing that the role of the hospital is one of rehabilitation rather than custodial care, unfortunate reactions are avoided which are generated in a patient when sent to a closed hospital, frequently after some minor misdemeanor, which he regards as resulting in an unfair form of imprisonment.

Training for Community Living

One cannot start to rehabilitate patients back into society satisfactorily until one breaks away from the conventional idea of occupational therapy as a means of occupying the patient with little thought of its actual value in relationship to work outside. The first step is to get away from the idea of one person producing one end product, for with subnormals this immediately leads to difficulties. What are really required are good work habits in the patient together with some degree of adaptability. Poor time-keeping, irregular output, and failure to ask for advice when in difficulties, are all factors which cause subnormals to lose jobs in the community and therefore require tackling while the patient is in hospital. At Ladysbridge, considerable use is made of incentive payments in relation to both work and behavior. These are coupled with the further incentive of full parole outside the hospital, which is looked upon as a great step toward returning to the community and therefore highly valued.

Patients work in teams. Males are employed in coal briquette production and making concrete paving slabs, curb edgings, etc., together with a considerable quantity of woodwork of the assembly variety. One is always left with a well-finished, salable article. "Sales of work" have been stopped and articles are only produced that have an economic value and can be sold commercially at a small profit. There are four months' advance orders for woodwork all the year round, orders for at least 1000 paving blocks at any time, and regular orders for coal briquettes with a turnover of about 90,000 a year.

Patients working on these schemes are assessed by the nurses in charge of the group on a points system which covers regularity of work, output, and quality. Patients are paid at the end of the week on the number of points gained. The maximum of 7½ points earns 15 shillings ($2.10). Attached to this incentive scheme is another called "attitude" which covers all aspects of the patient's behavior considered socially unacceptable. Here the patient starts with a total of 5 points and loses points over the week for behavior deemed socially incorrect. For instance, frequent swearing, going around in a state of partial undress, persistent fighting, or any behavior leading to group disharmony is likely to lose points. Achievement of 75 per cent of the maximum points from both scales automatically entitles parole. Patients are paid on normal community pay days by wage packet with the figure noted on the outside as they would be if working in the community. The idea of building up savings from a basic salary is stressed, money being deducted from wages and banked in their own accounts. Patients are encouraged to spend savings to buy their own clothes, transistor radios, watches, etc. Going into shops and purchasing articles on their own initiative is essential if they are to manage at home.

Girls are rated on similar scales and the majority are trained in domestic work. It is essential to ensure familiarity with domestic appliances usually found in homes, such as electric irons, kettles, vacuum cleaners, washing machines, etc. Unfamiliarity in a domestic situation might cause tension, with subsequent breakdown. For example, one patient said she had been sacked because "Mrs. — doesn't like me." This was checked and found to be untrue. On questioning, the patient said she was unable to use a vacuum cleaner and was afraid to ask how lest she show her ignorance. She attempted to deal with the situation by a complete change of job and the hope of a different kind of cleaner at the next house.

When ready, both male and female patients are found jobs in the surrounding area, travelling daily between hospital and work. Conversely, day patients are admitted from the surrounding area, who are unsuitable for employment outside, but who can work in one of the hospital departments. They live at home, travel daily to the hospital, and are paid for their work. One 14-year-old girl travels 43 miles daily to make use of this service. Parents put them on the bus and a nurse meets them at a stop adjacent to the hospital. In the evening the nursing staff see them onto the correct buses and they are met by their parents upon arrival.

Faulty dental hygiene is often a cause of considerable upset and pain with subsequent behavior disorder in mental defectives. Parents, therefore, whose children are troubled with this problem, are assisted by admitting the children overnight, having them seen by the hospital dentist, and returning them to their homes the following day.

Group psychotherapy with groups of eight to ten subnormal patients is practiced on both male and female wards. Specific subjects tend to be discussed such as problems involved in working outside the hospital, relationships between punishment and behavior in hospital and community, relations with the opposite sex, and so on. Progress was slow at first due to feelings of insecurity but now patients verbalize their problems much more freely. This has tended to reduce aggressive behavior among those who frequently used this outlet for their tension. Patients who have failed at work are brought into the groups and the causes of their failure discussed by their ward-mates. The fact that many of a subnormal's problems are due to lack of simple information is often brought out and can then easily be corrected. Further education classes are conducted by a psychologist and the chief male nurse, and considerable expansion in this field is anticipated.

Conclusion

These then are some of the ways in which the mental deficiency services are attempting to play their part in the overall scheme of community mental health in northeast Scotland. It is clear that mental deficiency is as much a community problem as is mental illness. Seen in this way the integration of the social services toward improving the welfare of the defective becomes of paramount importance. While there is no prospect of remedial treatment, rehabilitation by training must be a combined enterprise by many agencies in both the hospital and community.

CHILD PSYCHIATRY

Child psychiatric services in the region lag considerably behind the services offered to adults, reflecting the situation in Scotland as a whole.

A small outpatient service was begun at the Sick Children's Hospital in 1937. Though the staff were well trained, facilities at the hospital severely limited progress for over twenty years. Even after the introduction of the Health Service, financial priorities prevented any further expansion. This was mainly due to the fact that child guidance had long been regarded as primarily an educational responsibility. Government grants were accordingly more generous for education than for health authorities. However, it is paradoxical that, while other aspects of the mental health service were expanding, so little was done to develop so crucial an area as child psychiatry.

This relative stagnation of child psychiatry was partially relieved when, in 1950, the newly opened child guidance center of the local education authority provided facilities for active cooperation between educational psychologists and psychiatrists. In 1961, the hospital authority appointed its first consultant in child psychiatry and made provision, in a large new outpatient building, for a greatly enlarged department.

At present, the staff comprises a full-time psychiatric social worker, a half-time clinical psychologist, and a half-time secretary. One hundred and fifty patients below the age of 12 are referred each year. An inpatient unit for ten children with day patient facilities for a similar number is now being planned. By 1966 fuller treatment facilities will be offered and teaching potential for medical and other staff will be improved.

It now seems possible to make more rapid progress in the provision of an adequate service linked in with the other established and developing mental health services.

In-service Training

It is evident that teaching and the dissemination of the insights of child psychiatry must constitute a high priority for the new department.

Case conferences are the best introduction to the field for interested staff. After participation in case conferences some practitioners gain further experience through in-service training. This consists of supervised treatment of selected cases in collaboration with the psychiatric social worker dealing with the parents. This classic, child psychiatric approach forces the trainee to face the anxieties involved in the treatment situation and to learn to listen for the meaning behind the communication. It is thought to be superior to more formal teaching and also to "giving experience" by exposing the trainee to more numerous diagnostic interviews.

Such in-service training is offered to psychiatrists in training, school medical officers, and pediatric trainees with the object of enabling the doctor to take on a fuller role in his own field. The psychiatrist will be more conscious of his patients as members of a family and recognize their importance as parents. The school medical officer familiar with the child psychiatric service can make the mental health of schoolchildren his concern and offer valid advice to teachers. In the infant welfare clinic the same medical officer will be alert to the earliest insecurity of the nursing couple and offer more than a "change in formula." The pediatrician, in whose practice emotional difficulties are commonplace, will be less prone to offer simple reassurances on the basis of negative physical investigations and will be more skilled and confident in exploring the basic problems.

At present only one session a week is available for in-service training because of lack of space, but it is hoped to accept two or three trainees in the new outpatient department. The time spent by clinic staff on this scheme may detract from the present service capacity of the department but should pay dividends in community health in later years.

Interdepartmental Cooperation

Of similar importance are clinic contacts with a wide range of social agencies concerned with the destinies of children. In the care of children's officers in this region are about 1500 children, many of whom have been exposed to traumatic situations. An unknown number are seriously affected by their experiences, reflected in the fact that 15 per cent of clinic referrals are instigated by children's officers. These children are often less in need of specific psychiatric treatment than of a total therapeutic environment. The purpose here must be to give those responsible for the care of the child an understanding of the dynamics of the situation so that they can avoid being driven along the path of a past trauma by the child's blind repetition compulsion. Equally important, the child's present limitations must be respected if he is to fulfill his ultimate potential. To make excessive demands on a child's limited responsiveness rouses his anxiety and leads to a further impairment of his relationships. The mere recognition and acceptance of such limitations by those in charge can be a major therapeutic achievement and the turning point in a child's career. These aims are achieved by working with the foster parents, often accepting that the child's attendance at the clinic is only a means of bringing the foster parents into the treatment situation. Children in institutions are best seen in their usual surroundings so that the staff can be drawn into discussion of the problems.

The infant welfare services offer scope for preventive work so far hardly explored. The training offered to medical officers has been mentioned, but it is of equal importance to offer insightful experience to the health visitor who is in a unique position to gain the confidence of the mother and her infant during home visits and to detect the earliest signs of tension in the relationship of the nursing couple. It is not possible to make case material available to health visitors for training, even though over one-fourth of the patients are under six years of age. It may be possible to give health visitors more intimate contacts with child psychiatric methods once inpatient and day patient services are available. In the meantime, participation in case conferences at the clinic and a health visitor group, led by the psychiatric social worker, discussing problems from the health visitor's own experience seem the best modes of inducing her to take a wider view of her role.

Clinic Intake and Treatment Processes

Shortage of staff led to modification of both intake procedure and treatment approaches. The psychiatric social worker visit as first contact was felt to be wasteful in time and it has become the practice for the psychiatrist to examine the parents and the child at the first interview. At first parents and child were examined separately but more recently a joint interview has been found to be more profitable. It is left to the parents to decide who will bring the child. Both parents attended in 18 out of 100 new referrals, the mother generally attending in the remainder.

The joint intake interview is the obvious procedure where young children are concerned. Toddlers should not be expected to leave their mother with any stranger. This is also forced upon one when a patient with separation anxiety hides physically behind mother. It is clinically useful to regard most of the problems of toddlers in terms of their attachment to mother. It can be seen as an over-attachment which is an anxious exaggeration of the normal clinging stage, or a lack of attachment which is a failure to develop the clinging stage, or forced denial of the frustrated need to cling (manic defense). On the whole, one feels happier about the toddler who anxiously clings to mother and whose potential neuroticism is foreshadowed in an ambivalent relationship to mother, than about the one who cheerfully leaves mother for toys and a stranger, whose problems are likely to be engendered by a lack of mothering and apt to lead to a personality disorder. While the problems of older children cannot be presented along such simple parameters, the quality of the mother-child relationship remains the most important of all the factors to be elicited in the first interview, and in the joint interview this is observed directly.

Most mothers are capable of a discussion of their problems in the presence of the child—many take it as natural, having followed this procedure with the general practitioner and pediatrician. Many children will be able to partake actively while all reveal something of their attitude to their parents. It is quite feasible to ask the parents to leave when this type of interview fails to be productive of more than a frozen exposition of the complaint by the parent. One finds the child more easily accessible in the knowledge that the psychiatrist accepts uncritically his terrible secret—soiling, stealing, failure at school, or whatever. One is almost universally surprised to find the parents on return more open and capable of constructive discussion.

This relaxation on resumption of the joint interview is a sufficiently constant phenomenon to merit further attention. It plays an important part in the success of this procedure by giving it the therapeutic import without which any "diagnostic" technique is meaningless.

FAMILY THERAPY. Parallel with the adoption of the joint diagnostic interview, the scope of treatment has been widened by adopting a family therapy approach. This is not, of course, a novel procedure, yet its formal acceptance arouses anxieties in the therapist who must abandon the secretive one-to-one relationship and lay bare his therapeutic skills, such as they are, to the criticism of the family. These anxieties are perhaps lessened if the first interviews are regarded as a continuation of the diagnostic interview. If at any time the individual needs of the child or his parents are revealed to be beyond the capacity of family treatment, the psychiatric social worker is drawn into the situation and treatment is continued along classic lines. This is so in the majority of cases taken on for treatment. It is felt, however, that the more intimate knowledge of the family situation conveys a considerable advantage to individual treatment. It is thus of little import that no precise indications for family versus individual therapy can be laid down at present, the main criterion for the adoption of family treatment being its early success, as evidenced by change within the family.

Observing family activities one notes a lessened focusing on the symptoms of the child and a redistribution of responsibilities within the family so that it approximates more the sociocultural ideal and, concurrently, the assumption of roles more appropriate to the real status of the family members. An early change in anxiety direction occurs frequently, e.g., a shift of focus from the delinquent child to the underlying family pattern of nagging, distrust, and apprehension. Concurrent with this acceptance is a lessening of the helpless feeling of being at the mercy of the child's "badness"; hence a lessening of anxiety.

By contrast, failure on the part of the therapist to effect change in the family pattern is evidenced by continuous circular discussions of the causes of the child's misbehavior, an insuperable resistance to interpreting the offending child's behavior in terms other than heredity, his badness, or at any rate his "nature." One cannot achieve a shifting of attention from the child's symptoms and these remain unchanged or deteriorate. The therapist soon finds himself clutching at straws—pathetic little reports of "I have been good" by the child who finds himself drawn to acting-out in a role which was not of his own choosing. It is then appropriate to change the treatment to individual therapy, often with rather limited prospects of success.

DRUG THERAPY. Any discussion of treatment would be incomplete without specifying the use made of drugs. In the past, the argument against drugs was clinched by their relative inefficiency, and resisting "symptom removal" converted pharmacologic impotence into a virtue. Now that drugs are more effective and symptom removal is a possibility for selected cases, it is opportune to restate the question whether or not symptom removal is harmful.

Drugs, usually Atarax in doses of 10 mg. three times daily, were used with 23 out of 100 children, and analysis of the 12 failures proves illuminating. In seven of these the drug was not administered either because the parents were unable to persuade the child to take it (three), the child was removed from home (two), or the parents could not face the prospect of seeing the object of their hostility improve (two). The remaining five failures included two children with school phobia and severe personality disorder with whom no therapeutic relationship was possible, one encopretic who improved unrelated to drug treatment, and one schizoid boy of ten whose failure was expected. The fifth was a child in local authority care who was counted as a failure since he did not respond before the study ended. Both parents and children defend very successfully against the threat of drug-imposed change. They do not need a concept of "symptom tolerance" to defend them. Where it is felt that a symptom, such as enuresis, is of current value to the child, one refrains from attacking it by drugs or "deconditioning," since the child will certainly find ways to defend the symptom effectively.

On the other hand, 11 children of the 23 receiving drugs definitely improved. In three of these, organic factors were considered important, and one proved to be epileptic. Atarax helped a mute motherbound child to tolerate the initial anxiety of therapy. Most of these children showed somatization of anxiety as a prominent feature; in five children, school phobia precipitated referral and the drug helped a quick return to school. Outside the organic syndromes the major indication for drugs is thus crippling anxiety, and drugs can be of definite help in psychotherapy, enabling the child to face what might have been an intolerable situation. Sometimes drugs will successfully remove a residual symptom, such as an enuresis, that has outlived by years its regressive purpose. Sometimes drugs will afford that slight relief in family tensions required to initiate treatment. Psychiatric anxiety regarding drugs will resolve if they are regarded not as a substitute for psychotherapy or as a short cut to a "cure," but as part of the total treatment plan.

Inherent in all drug treatment is the assumption that the developing child will benefit from relaxation of tensions, whether produced by drugs or other means, whether initiated in the child himself or in another family member. The other important application of drugs is thus as an aid to the treatment of the parents. Of 100 cases, five mothers and one father received drug treatment at the suggestion of the child psychiatrist, a ratio which may only reflect the greater number of mothers attending. The condition treated by drugs is usually a depressive illness, sometimes puerperal in onset, sometimes dating to a bereavement, usually of sufficient persistence to have had a detrimental effect on the children. A much greater number of mothers reveal a past history of depression which must have had causal effect in their child's disorder. It is to be hoped that in the future general practitioners and welfare staff will be sufficiently alerted to maternal depression so that the child victims of this condition will not need psychiatric attention because of it.

Conclusion

This brief account of the limited child psychiatric practice in the region must be seen against the background of extensive social services of other types for children, some of which have been described in this book. The dissemination of child psychiatric insights throughout this complex will be a long and arduous task, but the effort will both facilitate cooperative integration and be enhanced by it.

ALCOHOLISM

The World Health Organization defined the alcohol drinker in the broadest way by saying that heavy drinking should be regarded as drinking more than the culture permits, whereas the term *alcoholism* should be used to describe heavy drinkers in whom alcohol is, or shows prodromal signs of, impairing mental or physical health, or social or economic functioning. However, one must not lose sight of the possibility that heavy drinkers may drift into alcoholism.

The purpose of disease classification and diagnosis is to delineate a symptom complex so that when people talk about it they talk about the same thing; i.e., they can communicate about it. It enables people to recognize the symptom complex, to discover its natural history, and to experiment with its treatment, and so to make prognostications. The WHO definition is too broad to be useful for these purposes.

Jellinek (2, 3), after an extensive study in different parts of the world, has recently proposed a classification of alcoholism which is an advance in clarity. He avoided confusion with old terminology by labelling his divisions by letters of the Greek alphabet. In this region it has been found possible to ascribe most cases to one of Jellinek's groups.

The Size of the Problem
in Northeast Scotland

In the year from March 1, 1960, there were 73 new referrals for alcoholism to the psychiatric services, of whom 5 were females. Thirteen males and one female were seen only once, seven males and three females were treated as outpatients on more than one occasion and the rest were admitted either to the mental hospitals or to the regional mental health center. Of the 73 referrals, 20 came from the city of Aberdeen and 53 from the rest of the region.

There is little doubt that the number of referrals by no means represents the size of the problem. Probably it more closely relates to the facilities offered. There has been no field survey in the region which can throw any direct light on the number of alcoholics in the community. If Jellinek's indirect method is applied (5), using his values for the constants P (percentage of deaths from cirrhosis attributable to alcohol) and K (percentage of deaths from cirrhosis among alcoholics with complications alive in a given year), and the Registrar General's figures for deaths from cirrhosis of the liver in the region for the years 1955–1961 inclusive, 923 male alcoholics with complications or about 3000 male and female alcoholics with and without complications might be expected to be alive in any one year in this region.

This is startlingly different from the annual number of referrals and such numbers would certainly swamp the existing services. Yet, at 900 per 100,000 adult population, it is not a high rate as compared with estimates similarly obtained for other Western countries. The equivalent rate in 1948 for England and Wales was estimated to be 1100 and for the U.S.A., 3950.

It is recognized, however, that estimates by the Jellinek formula depend upon many unconfirmed assumptions and may therefore be considerably wide of the mark. Estimates from mental hospital admissions and other indirect methods suggest a larger alcohol problem in Scotland than in England and Wales and one which is rapidly growing. The male first-admission rates in 1961 in Scotland were four to five times higher than in England and Wales (incomplete figures), and from 1956 to 1960 the admission rates have doubled both in Scotland and in England and Wales (4).

Facilities for Alcoholics

There are no special facilities in the region at present for the treatment of alcoholics. Very few indeed of those who presented in 1960–1961 were treated as outpatients. It is the experience here that by the time an alcoholic is persuaded to come for treatment he usually requires a period as an inpatient. If so, he goes to the admission ward of one of the mental hospitals. Rather few alcoholics are referred to hospital via routine psychiatric outpatients. They come straight from their general practitioner, from the psychiatric emergency service centered on the Ross Clinic, from various voluntary bodies, and from general hospital departments. Some are self-referred.

The Practice at the Royal Mental Hospital

A large majority of alcoholics admitted are males and go into the male admission ward, which took 215 general psychiatric admissions in 1962. The ward is staffed by one part-time consultant devoting nominally only four sessions a week to it and full-time assistant physicians varying considerably in skill and experience, sometimes from overseas with the expected difficulties in communication and cultural empathy, and varying in number between three at the most and more often only one. They have other extensive commitments in the chronic wards of the hospital. A fractional share of one psychiatric social worker is all that can be claimed. There are three qualified nurses, only two of whom are on duty at the same time, and three assistant, or student, nurses.

Treatment is essentially eclectic, each case being judged on its merits. There is no rigid period of stay in the hospital. The disadvantages of losing a job have to be weighed against the possible advantages of a longer sojourn in hospital, especially when there is an appreciable degree of unemployment. Whatever the treatment, the period in the hospital serves to withdraw the patient from alcohol fairly certainly, to subject him to the group environment, and to introduce him to Alcoholics Anonymous. The attitude of the staff is largely permissive. It is made clear that the decision to remain in hospital rests primarily with the patient. If he is determined to leave, he is not greatly pressed to stay since in this way a better long-term relationship will be established and so, should he relapse, it is hoped that he will more readily return.

On admission there is a full physical examination and any relevant investigations are performed, although only the Wassermann reaction is routine. A full psychiatric history is taken and, where possible, corroboration is sought from a relative or friend.

Treatment Techniques

MILIEU THERAPY.   In some patients the primary need is removal from the situation which has provoked recourse to alcohol and in which alcohol is readily available. It may be that no more specific therapy is required than participation in the ward routine with its one group meeting a week, occupational therapy, ward work, and social activities.

DRUG THERAPY.   Drugs may be employed in the following ways:

1. To control withdrawal symptoms (tremor, agitation, delirium), chlorpromazine or haloperidol are the drugs most commonly used. Up to 1000 mg. of chlorpromazine or 20 mg. haloperidol, by mouth or parenterally per day, are usually sufficient.
2. To treat the underlying anxiety states or depressions, tranquilizers or antidepressant drugs may be used.
3. To deter from a return to drinking, disulfiram is used but not routinely. Some patients have made the plea that it was lowering to their morale to feel dependent on some other "drug" in place of their alcohol. In many cases this is a resistance, but a

few patients seem to do well without disulfiram. Where it is used, a test dose of alcohol is not usually administered because in some cases it has been found to be much less unpleasant than the patient expected so that the deterrent effect is considerably reduced.

4. To correct malnutrition. If heavy drinking has interfered with food intake, vitamins are given in full dosage, parenterally in the first week or longer if necessary.

PSYCHOTHERAPY. All patients in the ward, including alcoholics, take part in a nondirective group meeting once a week. At present there are no special groups for alcoholics conducted by a physician experienced in group psychotherapy. Individual psychotherapy is very largely supportive and advisory in nature. More intensive, analytically orientated, individual psychotherapy is very seldom practiced. Time for it could only be found by the existing staff at the expense of some other endeavor, and it is doubtful if the results with alcoholics would justify this sacrifice.

AVERSION THERAPY. Apomorphine in 6 mg. doses has been used here to produce vomiting following the taking of alcohol in the treatment situation. Three administrations per day on five alternate days have been the course employed.

Obviously almost endless variations in technique could be devised and many have been described. In principle it is hoped to create an association in the patient's mind between the drinking of alcohol and something unpleasant, thus promoting a distaste for drink. However, it seems naive to imagine that a short and superficial experience such as a course of aversion therapy as usually practiced, would change for long such a well-established and probably deep-rooted behavior pattern as that of drinking alcohol. Experience with behavior therapy in the treatment of some of the neuroses has sometimes suggested that the newly learned behavior is limited to the treatment situation and that there is very little generalization.

In the last half-century, political fanatics have resorted to in-human and degrading techniques of brainwashing, embracing all forms of physical and mental torture, in order to change attitudes and deeply held beliefs. Aversion techniques have a disquieting resemblance in principle to some of these. There is something unpleasantly punitive about them. It is doubtful if an ordinary psychiatrist, with a philanthropic approach to his fellow men, could countenance an aversion technique drastic enough to be effective.

COMPULSORY TREATMENT.   Under what circumstances should one compel an alcoholic to have treatment? How much right has the individual to free choice? How really free is his choice and how much is he the victim of his genes and his nurture? Should somebody who wants to drink heavily to the detriment of health and wealth be allowed to do so? Has the community any right to stop him? There would certainly be no public support in this country for the compulsory prevention of cigarette smoking despite the very strong statistical evidence suggesting that it leads to bronchial carcinoma.

The Mental Health (Scotland) Act, 1960, makes provision for the compulsory detention of people suffering from mental illness and leaves room for very broad interpretation. The nearest relative, or a mental welfare officer, if a relative is not available, makes an application based on recommendations by two doctors and approved by the Sheriff. The two doctors are required to state that in their opinion (1) the patient suffers from mental illness which, (2) requires or is susceptible to medical treatment, and is of a nature or degree which warrants detention in hospital for such treatment; and (3) that the health or safety of the patient or the protection of other persons cannot be secured otherwise than by such detention. The case is reviewed by the psychiatrist in charge of treatment during the fourth week of detention, and if the interests of the health or safety of the patient can now be secured in other ways, he is discharged from detention.

In applying these provisions to alcoholics the first question to be faced is: When is alcoholism a mental illness? This is a thorny problem and different people will answer it differently. Alcoholics Anonymous places much emphasis on their belief that alcoholism is an illness, but this cannot be accepted without reserve. Few people would question that the patient suffering from delirium tremens is acutely ill mentally, and could be properly detained against his wishes for treatment, which would certainly be required and would probably be effective. But patients in delirium tremens are usually beyond argument and will simply accept hospitalization without demur. Thus the immediate interests of health can be secured without detention.

At the other end of the scale, the heavy social drinker, even with cirrhosis of the liver, may well be in perfect command of his faculties and it is difficult to see why, if he wants to drink himself to death, he should be prevented from doing so. The borderline between a heavy drinker and an early addict to alcohol is none too easy to draw. When the amount of alcohol taken has slipped beyond the voluntary control of the individual, there seems reasonable ground for considering him to be ill and to qualify for detention under the Mental Health Act, though whether he is "susceptible to medical treatment" is again debatable.

In fact, compulsory powers are rarely used in this region. In the year from March 1, 1960, only two patients out of the 73 presenting were compelled to have treatment.

OUTPATIENT FOLLOW-UP. If geography permits, the discharged inpatient is seen at regular intervals. It is uncertain to what extent this has therapeutic value; time available for seeing these outpatients limits the scope of the encounter to a brief enquiry as to progress and a word of encouragement or advice. The continued surveillance may, nonetheless, remind the patient that his condition is serious and give him a short-term goal to remain sober until the next appointment.

Community Services

GENERAL PRACTITIONER. The general practitioner is usually the first to be consulted about any problems of alcoholism. It is through him that nearly all patients are first referred to the hospital service and to his care that all patients are returned on discharge. The degree of liaison between the general practitioner and the individual hospital practitioner is a personal matter. From the Royal Mental Hospital a full report, including a statement about prognosis and suggested courses of action in the event of a relapse, is sent when a patient is discharged. In some cases it is useful to speak to the general practitioner on the telephone while the patient is in the hospital. In this way valuable information about the home background to which the patient will be returning can often be obtained. Some general practitioners show much more patience and understanding with alcoholics than others. Those who have little time for them can hardly be blamed; relapses are too frequent to derive much moral satisfaction from the inordinate amount of time which can be spent over them and in the present structure of remuneration there is certainly no financial incentive to do so. But if a general practitioner has a special interest in the problem of alcoholism he can sometimes be of special help, particularly to the families of alcoholics, to whom much more attention could profitably be given.

LOCAL HEALTH AUTHORITY. Local authority health visitors see all patients discharged from mental hospital to the country districts. They are visited as a routine, a few weeks after leaving hospital, and a progress report is sent to the hospital. However, this service is mainly an information-gathering device and has only doubtful therapeutic value to the alcoholic patient. There are no other local authority services specially for alcoholics.

ALCOHOLICS ANONYMOUS. The Aberdeen branch of this worldwide association of men and women who recognize that they have a problem in alcohol, wish to stop drinking, and to help others to do so, was started in 1951 by two local alcoholics. The group meets once weekly and since its inception over 360 people have come seeking help. Of these, ten men and one woman attend the weekly meetings regularly and are sober. About fifty more are sober and in fairly regular touch but do not attend the meetings. About one-hundred have more or less broken off from A.A. but are also thought to be sober. Approximately two hundred are known to be drinking or have completely lost contact. Three men and one woman are active workers in the group. In 1954 the Aberdeen branch started a splinter group in the Royal Mental Hospital which meets once a week on a different evening from the parent branch. This meeting is attended fairly regularly by six sober outside members and serves to introduce any alcoholic patient in the hospital to A.A. It is estimated that perhaps one-fifth of these patients take a further serious interest in A.A. In 1957 another group was started at Elgin by ex-patients from the Royal Mental Hospital.

Early in 1962 a prisoner in Peterhead Prison asked the Aberdeen group of A.A. for help in forming a group of prison inmates. The governor of the prison and his staff have given their full cooperation to this project and the sanction of the Home Office has been obtained. The average attendance in 1962 was 10 members at each weekly meeting and rose to 15 in 1963. The group is only allowed to meet if one outside member is in attendance. No officer from the prison is present and this is considered to be a great privilege. It is impossible to maintain the anonymity of the members who visit the prison as their full names and addresses must be sent to the governor prior to the meeting and taken again at the gate by the officer on duty.

Besides the group meeting in the prison every week, the leader also has private interviews with individuals on personal problems such as marital relationships, psychological disturbances, perversions, and other mental health problems. Although the organizer is quick to point out that he only feels well qualified in problems of drink, he finds that the bond which is set up through the common problem of drinking may lead to a freer discussion of other problems. Psychiatric or spiritual help may then be brought in.

It has been claimed that A.A. succeeds where all else has failed, and indeed it may in some individuals. But to compare "success" rates for different forms of treatment is misleading and unjustifiable unless patients are allocated at random to the different treatment groups.

Improving the Present Services

Any changes in the existing services will almost inevitably cost money. It must be accepted that there is no immediate prospect of a breakthrough in treatment which would lead to strikingly better results. In the present state of knowledge there is really little to offer alcoholics in the way of psychiatric treatment, so that although there are probably large numbers who do not come forward for treatment, it would be unrealistic to take extravagant steps to persuade them to do so, and money spent in improving the facilities for their treatment should be proportional to the efficacy of the treatments available.

HOSPITAL SERVICES.   Alcoholics from the county go to the Royal Mental Hospital, those from the city to Kingseat Hospital, and a few from anywhere in the region to the Ross Clinic. It might be more economical in staff time to streamline the arrangements and have a single regional inpatient psychiatric unit for nothing but alcoholics. Patients in such a unit would be a homogeneous group and might mold themselves into a useful therapeutic community. It might be easier to persuade an alcoholic to accept admission to such a unit, than to go into an ordinary mental hospital ward. It would be easier to undertake research projects at such a unit than it is at present, when the alcoholics in the region are treated in a number of different places. Lastly, such a unit could act as a center from which to coordinate the community and hospital services.

COMMUNITY SERVICES.   It is possible that too much time is now spent in checking up on individual patient's activities in a profit-less way without much idea as to what one is going to do about what one finds. It might be more profitable in the long run if health visitors, psychiatric social workers, and other interested workers, were to spend more time in giving support to the hard-pressed wives and families of these patients. They often find it difficult to take into their confidence any neighbors, or even rela-tives, and they may derive great help from being able to discuss the difficulties with somebody who has some understanding of them, even if the practical situation cannot be much altered.

The prophylactic possibilities have been little explored. This is hardly surprising as so little is known about etiology. The only person likely to be in a position to advise potential alcoholics is the general practitioner, many of whom make every effort to warn a known heavy drinker of the dangers of becoming addicted to alcohol. Again, in some circumstances it is possible to advise a change of job when the drinking patterns expected in it are threatening to create an addict from a heavy drinker. However, this sort of counselling is merely scratching at the surface of the problem and until more is known about what genetic or environmental factors go to make addicts, there seems to be little more that can be done.

The kinds of data which may be of value have recently been published by McCord and McCord (5), in their very careful analysis of the Cambridge Somerville material which was collected from 1935 onwards. It forms the basis of a prospective analysis which has already shown that a number of social factors significantly predispose to alcoholism. Perhaps by the timely intervention of social service agencies in the future some embryo alcoholics may yet be aborted.

REFERENCES

1. Exton-Smith, A. N., Norton, D., and McLaren, R. *An Investigation of Geriatric Nursing Problems in Hospital.* National Corporation for the Care of Old People, 1962.
2. Jellinek, E. M. *The Disease Concept of Alcoholism*, New Haven, Conn.: Hillhouse Press, 1960.
3. Jellinek, E. M. Alcoholism, a genus and some of its species. *Canad. Med. Ass. J.* 83:1341, 1960.
4. Kidd, C. B. Criteria for admission of the elderly to geriatric and psychiatric units. *J. Ment. Sci.* 108:68, 1962.
5. McCord, W. M., and McCord, J. *Origins of Alcoholism.* Stanford, Calif.: Stanford University Press, 1960.
6. Morrison, S. L. Alcoholism in Scotland. *Health Bull.* 22:12, 1964.
7. Post, F. *The Significance of Affective Symptoms in Old Age.* Maudsley monograph, No. 10. London: Oxford University Press, 1962.
8. Richardson, I. M., Brodie, A. S., and Wilson, S. Social and medical needs of old people in Orkney. *Health Bull.* 27:1, 1959.

9. Robinson, R. A. The practice of a psychiatric geriatric unit. *Geront. Clin. Additamentum*, p. 1, 1962.
10. Royal College of Physicians of Edinburgh. *Care of the Elderly in Scotland.* Publication 22, 1963.
11. Wilson, L. A., Lawson, I. R., and Brass, W. Multiple disorders in the elderly. *Lancet* 2:841, 1962.
12. Woodford-Williams, E., McKeon, J. A., Trotter, I. S., Watson, D., and Bushbury, C. The day hospital in the community care of the elderly. *Geront. Clin.* 4:241, 1962.
13. World Federation for Mental Health. *Report on the First Session of the Alcoholism Subcommittee.* World Health Organization, Technical Report Series, No. 42. Geneva, Switzerland, 1953.

The Rehabilitative Process

It is not the purpose here to become embroiled in a semantic wrangle in search of any absolute definition of the term *rehabilitation*. The aim is to state some of its usual connotations and explore others in order to provide criteria against which to describe and examine the rehabilitative process in the northeast region.

Living in Western industrial civilization, it is not surprising that the medical rehabilitative goal has for long been equated with enabling the patient—after some accident, injury, or illness—to become a solvent, efficient economic unit capable again of earning his livelihood. This apparently materialistic aim for our fellowmen carries with it the implicit assumption that from this source stem also happiness, self-esteem, societal regard, and status. In this guise the rehabilitative goal entered psychiatry from general medicine and has survived relatively unchallenged until recent years.

Particularly in the last 20 years there has been increasing and more insistent questioning of this goal and the assumptions which underlie it, and whether it has the same relevance for the psychiatric patient as for his physically disabled brother. It is more and more appreciated that assumptions about the import and value of work stem from a middle-class value system which is not equally applicable to, nor central to all men. The spread of psychodynamic theory in psychiatry has also brought a deeper understanding of critical processes in the psychiatric patient which have relevance to his restoration. There has been a minimal shift from the con-

667

centration of concern with the rehabilitation of the chronic hospital patient to others whose illness may be less symptomatically devastating but whose community tenure may be equally precarious. Indeed, there is a growing tendency to deny any dichotomy between rehabilitation and treatment and to postulate instead an indivisible adaptation of the total man to his total environment, whether in sickness or health, whether in hospital, at home, or at work, as the primary focus of concern.

Yet there remains some acceptance of this dichotomy in the expression of psychiatric staff roles and service functions. Psychiatrists and nursing staff are broadly regarded as treating agents, with psychiatric social workers, occupational therapists, and some community-based agents having a primarily rehabilitative role. This does not deny that there is often role shift and role multiplication —indeed, one of the dilemmas in some professional groups is the conflict between their own perception of their role and the different role demands that are in fact made on them. The service facilities which are regarded as principally fulfilling a rehabilitative function are "after-care" services, foster care services, sheltered workshops, halfway houses, ex-patient clubs, and perhaps to a lesser extent day centers and night centers.

There is also a general concensus that certain goal areas of patient adjustment are properly part of the rehabilitative process. This excludes any direct intervention to assess or relieve psychological symptoms, but includes the following:

1. *Vocational adaptation.* This concept has been broadened and no longer occupies the exclusive and central position of the earlier economic model. It involves occupational assessment, training, and placement, but also concern for training or retraining the housewife in problems of family budgeting, meal preparation and planning, and household chores.

2. *Educational rehabilitation.* Here the concern is with preparation for the proper fulfillment of the individual's leisure life. It attempts to develop talents, curiosities, and special interests through participation in activities or direct instruction.

3. *Family rehabilitation.* It is now generally agreed that family interaction and attitudes are often powerful both in bringing a patient into psychiatric care and in threatening his security of community tenure on leaving service contact. In particular, it is increasingly appreciated that long before entering psychiatric care the patient has been embroiled in a drawn-out distorted inter-actional process within the family orbit. Sometimes this is in relation to other disturbed family members, but more often it is just a denigrating hostile response of relatives to his behavior culminating in pressures to extrude him from the family both physically and emotionally. Thus the patient enters psychiatric care with a confused social identity which has to be restored and he has to return to an intolerant family whose image of him must be changed, and whose hostility and suspicion toward him must be replaced by something beyond mere passive acceptance. This is a problem as much for the acutely ill as for the chronically sick.

It is perhaps restoration in this sense which occupies a central position in current thinking about rehabilitation. It requires a greater understanding of cultural mores and norms. Aspects of behavior other than instrumental performance are often more central to the value systems of many people. Psychiatry must use understanding of social values to guide decisions about what to change or direct in the patient's behavior and attributes, in order to make him more acceptable to himself and to his family.

4. *General social rehabilitation.* The problems of distorted inter-action, extrusion, isolation, and role confusion in the patient, all have their counterparts in his relationship with a social sphere wider than the family unit. The processes are the same and the rehabilitative needs are similar. The patient needs to relearn old, or learn new, social skills and find modes of demonstrating his social effectiveness in terms appropriate to the culture. There is also a place here for communication between psychiatry and the community, but not in such platitudinous terms as that the psychiatric patient is ill in the medical sense and needs the tolerance, understanding, and protection society gives to the physically sick and infirm. Society does not perceive the behaviorally disordered

in this light. What the community requires is a more realistic translation of the causes of disorder derived from psychiatric perception to those derived from its own perception, together with some reassurance that the patient can and will conform to the behavioral norms that the community has established.

5. *Patient role modification.* In addition to restoring the patient to a proper, responsible, social self-image there is a somewhat neglected but nonetheless important aspect of the role problem. When a patient enters a hospital he runs the risk of adopting and becoming dependent upon the value systems he finds there. He is likely to act and think according to the hospital stereotype of a "patient," particularly a "good patient." This tends to deprive initiative and to produce behavior of little relevance to social living outside the hospital, often culminating in the well-recognized "institutionalization" syndrome. Any effective rehabilitative program must seek ways of modifying this role problem, which has its seeds in the trained attitude of medical and nursing staff and in the problems of controlling large numbers of people within a single organization. It finds further support in pressures of other patients to make a newcomer conform to roles with which they feel comfortable and which he has little role strength to resist.

REHABILITATIVE SERVICES
Occupational and Art Therapy

In the mental hospitals there are fairly standard occupational therapy and, in some hospitals, art therapy facilities. The concentration of effort in both is directed more toward assessment and symptom treatment than to restorative goals. Both imply educational rehabilitation in the sense of awakening interests and developing supplementary skills. Occupational therapy also attempts to create or reawaken work habits and drive, although the media often have very little relationship to real life. Patients are sometimes given daily chores within the hospital, but these are usually menial, repetitive tasks which are more calculated to perpetrate the individual's distorted social self-image.

The Halfway House

The first halfway house in the region was opened in Aberdeen in April, 1962, with accommodation for 11 residents. The site is a family house in a semi-professional, residential district. It went through the almost universal hazards of local petitioning against it, but the opposition was neither strong nor concerted and affected neither the support of the local authority nor the determination of the mental hospital superintendent who was its chief architect. The house has come to be known by its emotiveless street number —"375."

The house was set up in response to increasing realization of the importance in rehabilitating mental hospital patients, of close contact with the community, and gradual introduction to independence. It was believed that certain patients need a chance to seek work and have secure jobs before actual discharge. Some have to seek suitable accommodation before discharge is possible. The house was also designed to offer experience of circumstances as close as possible to community life.

The house is an adjunct of Kingseat Hospital and is staffed and administered by the hospital through the Board of Management. Clinically it is a ward of the parent hospital. The staff consists of one permanent sister-in-charge, three other nurses from the hospital, a full-time cook, and a full-time cleaner. The clinical director of "375" is the deputy superintendent of Kingseat who, with a psychiatric social worker, runs a weekly psychotherapeutic group involving all the resident patients and staff group discussions. Other medical staff also visit and continue to treat their own patients. Hospital social workers help individual patients with work, lodgings, and financial matters.

The choice of patients is intuitive because the halfway house movement as a whole is not sufficiently established to offer any realistic selection criteria. Nevertheless, the kinds of factors which commonly tend to govern selection are social difficulties such as inability to get on with others or lack of confidence in attempting to do so. Cases are chosen in which there is expectation that the unit will be more successful and quicker than the parent hospital in effecting community return. It is believed that the long-term hospital patient is the most needful of, and suitable for, rehabilitative care in "375." Geriatric patients and those who may offend the social standards of the residential area, such as alcoholics, overt homosexuals, and patients of bizarre appearance or behavior are currently considered unsuitable.

Residents are encouraged and helped to seek employment since this is regarded as the principal mode of community contact. There are few explicit rules of conduct and residents move freely in and out to seek and develop interests and relationships. They are also given complete freedom to invite anyone into the house.

Since the unit has only been functioning for a short period it is difficult to draw any conclusions about its general efficacy or its particular contribution to the rehabilitative process. There are few guiding principles available from the halfway house movement despite the proliferation of these facilities. To date, each halfway house seems to interpret, and perhaps achieve, something different from the diffuse goal of "providing a bridge across the gap between the hospital and the community." The architects of "375" are only too aware of the limitations of this model and the danger of accepting that provision of a service is necessarily equated with achievement of any definitive goal. With these strictures in mind a research program is being designed to detail and understand aspects of living at "375" which contribute to or impede achievement of rehabilitative goals. For example, the very close functional relationship of the house to the parent hospital may perpetuate the "patient" image in both residents and community. Although nursing staff do not wear uniforms, the reassuring hospital stereotype of attitude and approach may persist and foster authority dependence, making acquisition of an adequate social identity a slower and more difficult process. More must also be known about the community and family image of the house. The criteria for selection of patients may not be optimal, and it is only through research that one can be certain that covert forces do not operate to "select for success," unrelated to patient needs. Thus, the halfway house should be regarded as a pilot study of this mode of rehabilitation.

The Ashgrove Club

In return for contributing to the extended day center accommodation at the Ross Clinic, the Mental Health Association was given its use for a rehabilitation center operating in the evenings. The Ashgrove Club came into being in June of 1963, with a small management committee appointed from the association and consisting mainly of lay members with one junior hospital administrator and an educational psychologist. No medical staff have any direct participation in organizing or running the club. This exclusion is part of a deliberate policy toward creating a nontreatment atmosphere and a nonpatient image.

Membership is open to recently discharged, about to be discharged, or ex-hospital patients, and patients currently in outpatient treatment, recommended by any local psychiatric hospital or individual therapist. Members are of both sexes, and efforts have been made to limit the age range to about 25–45 years, although the possibility of starting separate club meetings for an older age group is being considered. Patients of subnormal intelligence are excluded. Final selection of members is in the hands of the committee, with provision for a short trial period before full membership is granted.

The general aim of the club is "to assist in the recovery of members in every way available to it, in particular:

1. By the provision of opportunities for social, recreational, and cultural activities within the club premises and beyond.
2. By encouraging members to participate in the development and administration of the club.
3. By fostering contacts with the wider community through helpers and invited visitors who have something to offer.
4. By supporting the efforts of members to take an increasing part in the work and leisure activities of their own community."

The Ashgrove Club has made a small, thoughtful beginning, meeting once a week. The activities program is unstructured with dependence on spontaneous development of interests. The atmosphere is informal with no explicit rules of conduct, although the committee may report a member's unexpected behavior to his therapist or hospital, the member concerned being made aware of what is being done.

At first small, the club is being built up by controlled stages. A formal effort will be made at the end of the first year to assess progress and to develop more extensive programs. It is thus very difficult at this stage to draw any conclusion about its part in rehabilitative processes, but it is a major step toward bringing the community, represented here by the local mental health association, actively into responsible cooperation in restoring the psychiatric patient to itself.

PERSONS AND PROCESS
The Psychiatric Social Worker

Within the psychiatric services the psychiatric social worker is a key individual who is not only directly concerned in the treatment process in terms of evaluating and reporting the social situation and crisis antecedents, but also has responsibility for translating treatment gains into community action.

The rehabilitative processes available to the psychiatric social worker depend broadly upon three features. The first is the patient's symptoms and the possibilities of their remission, which help determine his potential degree of self-adjustment. Second, the psychiatric social worker needs to know something of the capacity of the immediate family and community to accept and participate in the full realization of the patient's adjustment. Finally, the process may depend upon what other services and professional skills are available to assist.

Within this framework, rehabilitation can be described in three nonexclusive overlapping categories.

Reconstruction, where the principal aim is to help the patient achieve a radical change in his life and to help the community accept and participate in the change; the kinds of patient situations which may call for reconstruction are:

1. Brain damage, where there is loss of previous functional

capability which is often dramatic. The main problem here is to encourage family and employers to accept the loss realistically.

2. Senile dementia patients, who are often able to return to community life, but again with loss of financial capacity. Here one of the dangers is complete acceptance by the environment of total incapacity, affording the patient a sick, helpless role and militating against realization of residual capacity. Alternatively, complete and obdurate rejection by the family may create the need for permanent settlement in a community facility such as an old people's home.

3. The remitted long-term illness, where the patient may have to relearn community living from simplest shopping to re-establishing social relationships. A semi-protected environment, such as a halfway house, may be necessary which may also allow him to demonstrate gradually his social effectiveness to a doubting family.

4. Neurotic reaction, where the patient has to learn to control antisocial or unacceptable traits and to develop less used but more socially acceptable aspects of his personality in coping with day-to-day living. It is necessary here to help the family to accept fluctuating progress.

Repair of attitudes and family interactional structure, devastated by the patient's breakdown or deterioration as with:

1. Acute florid breakdown, where there is loss of family confidence in "knowing" the patient and inability to predict his behavior. There may be splitting of attitudes toward the patient, often attacking the entire structure of family relationships.

2. Slow, deteriorating illness where the patient's behavior has worn down the family's tolerance, so that there is reluctance to resume life with him after treatment. There is particular need here to understand the judgmental systems of the family before any change can be effected.

Reconciliation, where both patient and family must come to terms with inevitable characteristics of the patient's illness without denying the positive aspects of the situation, as with:

1. Chronic recurrent illness, where the periodicity is accepted, so that "spells" of illness take their proper place and do not overshadow the healthy periods. The requirement here is for flexibility of attitude by both family and patient.

2. Mental deficiency, where the reality that the patient has some latent abilities which can be utilized is accepted together with the limitations of the defects.

The psychiatric social worker is inevitably involved in all three types of rehabilitation and depends upon the availability of other community agents and facilities, their cooperation, and the achievement of coordination between them. In this region, coordination is mostly effected by informal personal contact. More than just an understanding of basic roles, personal contact allows a more detailed assessment of the strengths and weaknesses of community agents which may help or hinder the patient.

Mental After-care Officers

The role of community services as responsible agents for care of the mentally ill has become more clearly underlined and the need for coordination more clearly specified by the 1960 Mental Health Act. One result has been the training of local authority health visitors as mental after-care officers.

These officers have roles in both psychiatric services and the local authority, often indeed with offices in both facilities. In the psychiatric services they become an extension of existing treatment and rehabilitation organizations. Working closely with medical and psychiatric social worker staff, the unique contribution of the officers is in their link with, and knowledge of, community services; thus providing opportunity for direct, positive cooperation and coordination among all those involved in the care of the patient.

Nurses in the Role of
Community and After-care Agents

The number of personnel within the psychiatric services whose training is principally directed toward after-care of patients in the community has not kept pace with increased awareness of the need. Knowledge of community processes and problems is often lacking among staff fulfilling a "treatment" role in the hospital service. As an experiment toward filling both these gaps, Kingseat Hospital has introduced a scheme to give both senior and junior nursing staff some experience and guidance in domiciliary work and its problems. Two senior male nurses are fully participating in the rehabilitative program of some patients. There is indication that a strong relationship formed by a patient and a nurse on the ward can be utilized in the community for the benefit of some patients in some situations. This is particularly so for the individual who has considerable difficulty in establishing relationships and may need the crutch of the nurse whom he knows and trusts. Patients who have added physical problems may find reassuring the presence of a nurse who can fulfill the dual role of treatment and rehabilitative agent. Only time will tell how far this type of contact is beneficial and what dangers it may hold in perpetuating unresolved dependency beyond the walls of the hospital.

Voluntary Community Agents

Within the past few years some members of the local British Red Cross Society have become active visitors to mental hospitals. Lonely patients are now assured of regular interested visitors who strengthen contacts with the community.

As a result of interest stimulated by the local Mental Health Association and culminating in several courses of lectures on mental illness, a "League of Friends" was formed in 1961 for both large hospitals in the region, and the idea has since spread to many other hospitals. Volunteers visit their adopted hospital regularly in various capacities such as running the beauty parlor and library, visiting patients, and providing material benefits like bus tours, Christmas presents, shawls, and so on. The Women's Voluntary Service runs a canteen in one hospital for patients and their visitors.

CONCLUSION

This brief overview of persons and facilities associated with the rehabilitative process has been limited to the psychiatric service *per se,* and omits the tremendous contribution and involvement of the local health authority in this field. Because of the increasing interrelatedness of these two branches of the National Health Service, this account does not do justice to all work directed to the rehabilitation of the psychiatric patient. It is certain, too, that within the psychiatric orbit there are many facets and many individual contributions which have received scant attention in these pages or have been omitted altogether. Having said this, what conclusion may be drawn, and what comparisons may be made between current thinking about rehabilitation and the practical realization of these goals in the northeast?

In general, the picture is of small beginnings in a program of development which encompasses many aspects of restoration. The positive virtue of this situation is that these approaches are regarded as experimental—often indeed with some evaluative design woven into the structure. These precautions may be very necessary to avoid the pitfall, so frequently met in psychiatry, of launching large programs of service in a vacuum of ignorance, often to become monuments of failure. This is perhaps one occasion where traditional Scottish caution is a very positive asset.

There is a tendency for many of the facilities and persons involved in the *rehabilitative* process to be closely linked with the *treatment* service. For example, the halfway house is regarded as a ward of the hospital with nurses and attendant physicians playing principal roles. The ex-patient club uses hospital premises. This close association is likely to color negatively both the patient's development of a social identity and the attitude of community members toward demonstration of the patient's ability to function as an effective social organism. Many similar centers in the United States have become concerned about these problems and have clearly divorced this type of rehabilitative facility from the treatment facility, both geographically and in terms of staff function. While there are certainly some advantages in the conjunction of treatment and rehabilitation within one integrated service, one of the disadvantages is the hierarchical structure with its too great an emphasis on traditional medical values as against social and cultural values. This may be offset in the future as more nonmedical, qualified workers, trained in the social and psychological sciences, become available to add their own skills and insights to those medically trained, and to take over a measure of the overall responsibility for patient care. This division of responsibility, effected within a comprehensive service, would permit a stronger and more coherent development of the rehabilitative process, with agents such as the psychiatric social worker and occupational therapist broadening their roles and becoming central in a coordinated program of planning and theoretical development. Around this professional core could be integrated other workers, whose goal is the restoration of the patient, but whose current practice is often a duplication of effort and sometimes even an impediment to realization of a total plan for the patient. In these ways the modern concept of rehabilitation as part of a total process may gradually be realized.

Epilogue: The Future

It is impossible to foresee with accuracy the future requirements of a service. Further developments will clearly depend upon economic, social, and professional factors that are by their nature indeterminate. Nevertheless, existing trends and other relevant data form the basis of predictions and allow speculations on the directions that future organization may take.

All the evidence suggests that, as services are increased in number and variety, there will be a commensurate increase in the demand on them. Referral and admission rates, which have been steadily mounting, are likely to continue to rise for some time to come. Outpatient attendances are also bound to increase in line with recognition of the value of these clinics, particularly with respect to psychotherapy and counselling. There is also the possibility of a compensatory trend in the opposite direction as general practitioners with more skill and experience in handling minor psychiatric disorders gradually assume a greater degree of responsibility for their treatment.

The optimism that anticipates a major breakthrough in the treatment of mental disorder must be tempered by the caution that, in the foreseeable future, the time required for the care of a patient will not be significantly reduced. The era of psychiatric penicillin is still not at hand. All procedures will become more exacting, precise, elaborate, and time consuming, and will require more staff to carry them out.

The trend from institutional care to community care has become so deeply rooted in current thinking, in practice, and in legislation that it seems established for a long time to come. This will lead to a shift in manpower and other resources from hospital to community services which will be achieved both by the transfer of hospital psychiatrists to outpatient and domiciliary practice and by the recruitment and training of local authority staff in the mental health field. At the same time a greater burden will be placed upon the family doctor, who will require not only better undergraduate training in mental health, but also close and continued contact with experts to keep his skills up-to-date.

MENTAL HEALTH SERVICE PLANNING:
THE MODEL AREA CONCEPT

It is probably easier to make plans around a tangible structure, such as a hospital, than around such an elusive entity as the needs of a potential psychiatric population. In the past, within the National Health Service, the more striking advances have been recorded in bricks and mortar. The biggest of all planning operations undertaken by the Ministry of Health in London and the Department of Home and Health in Edinburgh has been in their respective "hospital plans."

One of the pitfalls of planning in this way is that buildings that are to be occupied five to ten years hence are designed on the basis of knowledge of present or past demand. A historic monument is erected rather than a challenging prophecy. Only a complete knowledge of total community need, together with a complete grasp of the range of therapeutic resources likely to be available, can give rise to the perfect plan. The impossibility of achieving this ideal demands a compromise solution. Such a compromise may be attained in the concept of the model area, in which additions to the service are planned piecemeal, with built-in evaluation in relation to the whole at each stage. For instance, if a new early treatment unit is set up to provide quick turnover, its effectiveness would be continuously evaluated, both in relation to the objectives it was designed to reach, and in terms of its effect on the utilization of other facilities in the service. In the light of this initial experiment, further additions would be made, again subject to continuous, careful evaluation. Models so evolved can then be generalized and applied in other areas. Planning along these lines is more rational, practical, and economical. It allows flexibility to meet constant change and avoids the "once and for all" phenomenon that so much bedevils hospital planning. Simple structural planning, however successful for churches, museums, and other public amenities, must be replaced by live functional planning for a growing and changing mental welfare service.

The history of psychiatry in this and other countries shows that, as the stigma lessens and barriers of ignorance break down, psychiatric skills become more readily available, both at an earlier stage in the morbid process and for the treatment of milder forms of illness. The problem presented by the patient now appears in the context of his home, or in his every day life and is no longer seen only in the context of the hospital. Classic syndromes, meticulously described in the textbooks of the last century and the early part of the present century, form a lesser proportion of the psychiatrist's work. Varied syndromes presenting in psychological, social, family, and medical contexts assume a more prominent place and must be tackled as far as possible within the human and material situations in which they occur. Often it is the situation rather than the individual that requires "treatment." For this reason, psychiatric skills must be available to the patient in his home environment. There seems to be little place in the future for inpatient units remote from the patient's home from which he must return to the unchanged morbid situation in which his illness originated.

These considerations point to the need for psychiatric units to serve comparatively small and well-defined catchment areas and for each unit to build up close functional ties with all local authority and general practitioner services in its area. In the northeast of Scotland, thought has recently been given to plans for future hospitals and it is likely that most new development will take place on the site of the Royal Mental Hospital whose main buildings, now well over one-hundred years old, are due for demolition within the next ten years. Current professional thinking suggests two distinct possibilities, each with its own attractions.

First, it is thought that a single regional unit with a number of subsidiary special units might be built, ultimately replacing all others except Bilbohall in Elgin. The attraction of this idea is that it would compare in size and grandeur with the adjacent general and special hospitals already on the Foresterhill site or shortly to be built. There would thus be created, on one large campus, a complete, balanced hospital community serving the entire region.

The second idea is to have several relatively independent units scattered over the Royal Mental Hospital site, each with its own catchment area and each with its primary relationships established with the various community mental health services. The former scheme is essentially hospital based, medically orientated, and probably "inward looking." It may perpetuate the concept of the institution overmuch. The latter scheme is community based, essentially social in orientation, and "outward looking," and is to be preferred for these reasons.

It would be necessary to plan for perhaps four new independent units. Two units would serve the city of Aberdeen, a third the west and northwest areas of the region, and a fourth the northern area. Bilbohall Hospital would continue to serve its own present catchment area. Each of the new units would serve a population of about 100,000. Each *basic unit* would have approximately 200–250 beds for short, medium, and long-stay adult psychiatric patients. Associated with each basic unit would be one or more *special units* for groups such as adolescents, psychopaths, alcoholics, and geriatric and psychosomatic patients. This would allow the staffs to have both general and specialized experience. The general field would be limited to the catchment area while the special fields would embrace the whole region. The special units would vary in size but might comprise an additional 300–500 beds depending on the size of the geriatric unit. The plan would provide for up to 1500 beds. It is by no means certain that these would completely replace the 1800 beds in the Royal Mental and Kingseat Hospitals, but a gradual run-down of Kingseat as new units come into operation would make possible any modification to the plan and perhaps lead to the addition of one more basic unit.

The basic inpatient units would be in separate buildings, but outpatient departments might be combined under one roof. Day patient services could be provided only for patients living within commuting distance of them and might therefore be attached only to the two city inpatient units and Bilbohall.

Admission procedures would be developed for such emergencies as acute psychotics, suicides, and other acutely disturbed patients. A single unit, closely related to the present casualty department of the Royal Infirmary, and organized on a 24-hour rota system would be the most economical in manpower and the most efficient from the point of view of disposal, teaching, and research.

Certain services might be common to all the units, such as sheltered workshops for long-stay patients, kitchens, cafeterias, recreation halls, and cinema. Laboratory services and other special investigative facilities would continue to be centered at the adjacent general hospital which already provides a regional service of this kind. Most specimens for laboratory investigation can now be readily despatched anywhere. Whenever necessary, patients can attend for special investigations and in general there is no over-riding argument in favor of surrounding psychiatric ward units with assessment laboratories as is the trend in general hospitals. While this plan is wholly compatible with the most rigorous organic investigation of patients who require it, there is no inter-ference with the aim of placing the patient in a realistic human therapeutic environment. Nevertheless, there is a number of patients in whom significant organic factors require intensive investigation within a general hospital setting where more elaborate facilities are available. It has therefore been recommended that ten beds should be allocated to "psychiatric investigation" in the Royal Infirmary extension plan. Admissions would be arranged from the various units in the psychiatric service and duration of stay is unlikely to exceed two weeks, allowing for approximately 200–250 admissions in a year.

These ideas will mature and be modified over the next few years and will be put into effect during the 1970's.

DEVELOPMENTS IN TRAINING

A new undergraduate curriculum is being planned in the medical school. Almost certainly there will be more opportunity for teaching community psychiatry in its broadest sense. The recently established department of sociology, together with the departments of social medicine and psychology, will play an increasing role in medical education. They will set the pattern for the medical care of the future which will be increasingly concerned with chronic illness and disability, early prevention by social action, and an appreciation of the psychological component in all illness.

Psychoanalytically orientated therapy has not flourished in Britain as it has in the United States. Few academic departments have taken psychoanalysis seriously and psychoanalysts themselves have remained outside the mainstream of psychiatry. There is little sign of change although here and there psychoanalysts have been appointed to hospital consultant posts, mainly in child psychiatry. In this region, with recent additions to the psychiatric staff of some who have had a certain amount of dynamic training, it has become possible to plan a course of psychotherapy to be offered by the university in October, 1964. If the venture proves successful and if a demand emerges, this will become a formal postgraduate course in perhaps two years. It is hoped that this will gradually improve the psychotherapeutic skills of regional staff as well as provide some training for those from other centers. By raising the standard of psychiatric practice in the region, it is probable that recruitment to the specialty will be augmented. A further attraction to the field may come from the increasing amount of social and epidemiological research in the department of mental health. Young graduates realize that today a period of experience in clinical, social, or basic research is an essential prerequisite to promotion, especially in the academic world, and most favorable opportunities are now provided by the university, the hospital board, and the Medical

Research Council, making it possible for the young clinician to take time out for research training.

The Training of Nurses

It will soon be possible for psychiatric nurses to have a shortened general training and for general nurses to have a routine period of psychiatric training as part of their general course. In this way a much more versatile corps of trained nurses will be available in the region, enabling more efficient deployment of their skills. It is hoped that this scheme of comprehensive and integrated training will ultimately extend to all units in the region.

The shortage of *clinical psychologists,* which is nationwide, can only be overcome by additional training centers. Some thought has been given to the provision of a course in clinical psychology to be run jointly by the university departments of psychology and mental health. This would be linked to the existing probationer scheme in the hospital service and would allow trainees to be employed on a modest salary while attending the course.

A similar plan is being considered for the training of *social workers* when the department of sociology is fully established. It is known that a large number of young people leave Aberdeen for centers in the south to undertake social worker training and that they do not return. Only a local training school can prevent this drift and improve recruiting. There is little doubt that an attractive program could be worked out for a limited number of trainees, some of whom would be drawn into the mental health service.

FURTHERING THE INTEGRATION OF WELFARE

Apart from questions of planning specifically mental health and welfare services, the future of welfare in the northeast region can be visualized as a process of gradually developing integrated services designed to meet the changing needs of society. While it is not possible to cover the whole range, some of the more promising areas where new ideas are already under review can be described.

The General Practitioner Service

The local branch of the College of General Practitioners has been most active in establishing good working relations with the mental health service and psychiatrists have participated in refresher courses for their members. The college is deeply concerned with raising the standard of general practice by improvements in the undergraduate curriculum. A university department of general practice is suggested, which would give particular attention to the problems of medical care within the community, as against care in hospital. The department of social medicine has been actively engaged in sponsoring this scheme. Through the medium of improved undergraduate and postgraduate training, therefore, it is expected that the mental health service will benefit significantly from the skills of good general practitioners.

In recent years the hospital authorities have considered various schemes for attachment of general practitioners to the hospital service. A few have held part-time posts in the mental hospitals and have proved their value. Certain hospital units may be wholly or partially accessible to general practitioners to investigate or treat their own patients. This movement is greatly to be welcomed in psychiatry. In the future—especially when the new and smaller units come into existence—general practitioners will be increasingly regarded as an integral part of a total mental health service working closely with psychiatrists in the treatment of their own patients in both hospital and community.

Local Authority Services

The future holds immense possibilities for further development of local authority services. All recent legislation and the present climate of public opinion point the way to considerable advances in this sphere. Several difficulties will have to be overcome. First, the geographical boundaries of local authorities are much smaller than those of regional boards and extremely uneven in population and resources. A large city authority, such as that in Aberdeen, has the wealth, facilities, and manpower to make a significant contribution while a smaller authority, such as Banff, can hardly be expected to provide the same range of services. The Department of Home and Health for Scotland is currently planning reorganization of local authorities to offset some of these difficulties. From the point of view of mental health, it would be useful if the geographical boundaries of local authorities and regional boards were the same. This is unlikely to be possible so that the problem of services to more remote areas will remain.

A second difficulty is finance. A few years ago a system of block grants to local authorities was instituted replacing the older system of earmarked grants. Unhappily, this occurred when the Mental Health Act was being introduced with its emphasis on the development of local authority services. It was made clear by the Department of Home and Health that no special earmarked grants would be made in respect of the proposed new developments, with the result that the new schemes had to compete with established services, already underfinanced from central funds. Hence, local authorities have been given no real incentive to promote new or ambitious schemes. The hospital boards have had to continue to carry the major burden, not only of the hospital services proper, but also of certain community services, such as day centers, hostels, domiciliary care, and follow-up. It may have been thought that community care would be a cheaper commodity than hospitalization but the reverse is likely to be true. This quandary now troubles the policy makers, so heavily committed to the new idea. It is not likely that local authorities will show much enthusiasm until specific finance is made available for a whole range of services and facilities for the mentally ill and the handicapped.

A third difficulty concerns trained staff. Those employed by the hospital authority have better conditions and are the highest paid while those employed by the local authority work under the poorest conditions and are the lowest paid. Recently this differential has been, if anything, widening and there is now public concern about remedying this anomaly. It is to be expected that people with an interest in psychiatry should look for posts in the hospital service since their salaries and conditions would be so much more satisfactory than in the local authority service. At present it seems that more value is attached to curative than to preventive medicine and this is reflected in the comparative backwardness of the social sciences in Britain. The government has recently set up a committee to investigate the position of research in this field and will probably recommend the creation of a social sciences research council. While this may eventually help to ameliorate the situation by raising the financial backing and status of the field and so increasing its manpower, the basic problem of imbalance between resources for prevention and treatment, between local authority and hospital authority, has yet to be faced.

Rehabilitation and resettlement, particularly of long-stay patients, will continue to exercise both local authorities and hospitals. There are those who advocate the wholesale discharge of all able-bodied psychotics who are capable of minimal work, the setting up of hostels, and the provision of sheltered workshops within the community. However, such studies as those of the Social Psychiatry Research Unit in London have revealed that, for chronic schizophrenia at least, community services do little to lessen either the severity of the illness or the burden on the patients' families. It may be that a more conservative policy will return and that the hospitals will have to extend their own provision of workshops and other occupational activities for patients so severely damaged that a return to the community would not be a boon to them or to anyone else. This should not conflict with plans for more active and energetic efforts to return patients quickly to the community whenever the active phase of illness is over and when treatment has been completed, but there will be patients who, after perhaps several readmissions, will require that type of sheltered life-situation under prolonged special care that only good mental hospitals can provide.

Dispersed Services in the Community

Some years ago it was thought that a series of clinics in the larger towns, such as Fraserburgh, Peterhead, Huntly, Elgin, and Keith, would serve a useful purpose. A clinic at Peterhead proved unsuccessful, both doctors and patients preferring referral to the clinic at Aberdeen where facilities were better and where more privacy could be secured. Only the clinic at Elgin has flourished as part of the new peripheral unit based on Bilbohall Hospital. One reason for the lack of demand for peripheral clinics is that the domiciliary service is so active throughout the region. This brings psychiatrist and family doctor together on the case and where there is an indication for continued treatment at home, it can be given by the doctor with a certain amount of psychiatric supervision.

Three types of problems could be dealt with more effectively by local services: patients who would benefit from day hospital treatment, those requiring long-term after-care whether or not they are fit for sheltered occupation, and certain mental defectives for whom continuous hospitalization is unnecessary. In general, there might be fairly simple services for these patients, the day-to-day care being given by interested general practitioners with some training but under the overall supervision of a consultant whose unit has links with the area.

If small community mental health centers providing these services are set up, they could become the focus for other types of community service such as counselling, screening of high risk groups, and registration of vulnerable individuals, all of which are desirable measures toward the ultimate aim of preventing breakdown. Social workers and specially trained health visitors or district nurses would integrate these mental welfare centers with the other social welfare services.

The General Hospitals

The trend in the northeast toward a self-contained mental health service with comparatively slender connections with the general hospital service is unusual at a time when general hospital psychiatric units are becoming the fashion, especially in England. However, the move away is more apparent than real, as this volume has tried to indicate.

Joint outpatient clinics and schemes for attachment of psychiatrists to general wards could be extended. This is much to be welcomed as additional staff becomes available. It is hoped that the general hospital service itself will become more outward looking as the proportion of chronic cases continues to increase and as the social and psychological dimensions of all disease become more apparent to the average hospital doctor. It is felt that the insights provided by those working in the field of mental health have much to contribute to medical practice as a whole.

Pediatrics

With the diminution of acute illness among children and the lessened need for hospitalization for the sick child, pediatrics has become increasingly concerned with "child health," particularly with child mental health and development. Child psychiatrists see here a problem in definition of the boundaries of their two disciplines. However, the disturbed or maladjusted child will remain the concern of the child psychiatric team, though the active cooperation of the pediatric physician is likely to be sought more and more. Joint clinics for the assessment of handicaps of all kinds are being planned and family counselling clinics may emerge from this cooperative effort.

The Penal System

The increased burden of psychiatric offenders which will be placed on the mental health services will demand reorganization to meet the special needs of these patients, many of whom are in the younger age groups and predominantly male. Psychopathic units may not completely meet the need unless there is provision within them for security. Although the problem in Aberdeen is less acute than in the larger cities, the experimental approach of the model area concept is particularly apposite in this kind of problem. Research is already planned to include a systematic investigation of the service needs of the psychopathic patient, and definitive service plans may eventually be evolved on this basis.

There is much else that requires to be done for those who exhibit antisocial tendencies as part of their mental disorder. It has been recommended that a consultant with special experience of forensic psychiatry should be appointed to the region, whose duties would include an advisory service to the courts, the police, the probation department, the approved school, and the two prisons. He would be responsible for the small inpatient unit at Peterhead Prison and would have charge of the psychopathic and other forensic beds in the new hospital plan. This would open up further opportunities for research and for improvements in the treatment of offenders.

NEW CONCEPTS

The experience of those working in mental health in the north-east region is probably very much the same as in other parts of the world. No unique features are claimed for this service except for the bringing together of as many established skills and insights as finance, material facilities, and manpower will allow. It is a logical consequence of the experience gained that increasing attention is now being paid to unsolved problems, the relevance of which is hard to appreciate in the daily round of clinical pressures, but which in the end become obstacles to clinical progress. The answers to such questions as identification of illness, classification of disease, prevalence, incidence, the natural history of mental disorder, and the relation between breakdown and the social and personal conditions leading up to it, form the premises from which all theory and practice follow. It is becoming increasingly apparent here as elsewhere that the differential perception of deviant behavior is a phenomenon of central importance in the process of breakdown and referral and that individual and group tolerances require as much study and treatment as do the internal malfunctions of the individual patient.

CONCLUSION

The central theme of this book has been the integrative character of the development of social and mental welfare. It is clear that the achievement of higher levels of total community welfare will necessitate the solution of problems obstructing even closer integration, such as have been described. Integration is a *sine qua non* of maximal community welfare.

Yet, with the burgeoning organization of welfare at every level of authority from the voluntary organization to the central government comes increasing power over individual, family, and community values. The more closely psychiatry is associated with the social aspects of welfare, particularly if it involves a movement away from the medical milieu, the more important it will be to heighten awareness of mental health and social goals. For instance, an understanding of the social processes involved in differential tolerance of deviant behavior may imply not only control over differential rates and distributions of morbidity, but also control over the social processes themselves. While such matters remain purely problems in scientific research there need be little concern for the consequences. But the application of new knowledge is always the ultimate social sanction for acquiring it, as the nuclear bomb bears witness, and the eventual outcome of understanding mental and social processes could be at least as potent. The concepts of *treatment, service, care,* and *welfare* are means which can be either instruments of constructive social change or weapons of cynical destruction. The community's right to self-protection can only be upheld by vigilance in relating them to socially accepted goals. The mental health worker, as the agent of social discrimination, perhaps more than any other in welfare, may be the key to achievement of new social objectives defined for him by the community of the future.

Index